PRACTICAL CHINESE QIGONG
FOR
HOME HEALTH CARE

Compiled by
Jin Ce Hu Zhanggui Jin Zhenghua

Translated by
Li Peijin Li Guangli

FOREIGN LANGUAGES PRESS BEIJING

First Edition 1996

ISBN 7-119-00070-5

© Foreign Languages Press, Beijing, China, 1996

Published by Foreign Languages Press
24 Baiwanzhuang Road, Beijing 100037, China

Distributed by China International Book Trading Corporation
35 Chegongzhuang Xilu, Beijing 100044, China
P.O. Box 399, Beijing, China

Printed in the People's Republic of China

Foreword

Qigong is a gem of traditional Chinese medicine. According to historical records, it has a history of nearly 3,000 years. It is a unique medical health care method which the ancestors of the Chinese nation gradually created, accumulated and organized during their cumulative lives and medical practice.

Traditional Chinese medicine holds that *yuanqi* (vital energy) is the root of life —the starting factor of life's growth and visceral activities. A human body's health situation depends on the degree of rise and fall of *yuanqi*: if *yuanqi* is plentiful, and viscera coordinated, one will be in good health; however, if *yuanqi* is insufficient or damaged, diseases may occur. Traditional Chinese medicine also considers the maintenance process of human bodies' normal life activities as a result of balance of *yin* and *yang*. Any imbalance of *yin* and *yang* may result in illness. Through exercise of body, breath and heart, Qigong cultivates and strengthens a person's *zhenqi* (*yuanqi* or *zhenqi*—vital energy). It helps retain the balance of *yin* and *yang*, clear and activate the channels and regulate *qi* and blood so as to prevent and cure diseases, keeping the body in good health. Modern medicine has proven that Qigong has some regulatory functions on the nervous, respiratory, digestive, circulatory and endocrine systems, and can promote the stability of internal circulation.

There are two ways to cure diseases using Qigong: the first is for a Qigong master to send external *qi* to patients; however, this kind of Qigong master is very rare. Also, curing disease by external *qi* greatly consumes a Qigong master's strength, thereby preventing him from meeting the needs of a great many people. The second is a self-treatment method. A patient can practise Qigong alone to improve physical functions, strengthen physique and rid the body of diseases. The Qigong introduced in this book belongs to the latter method. The book is called *Practical Chinese* Qigong *for Home Health Care* in order to emphasize that practice of these Qigong movements do not require a special location. They can be at home, a park, a courtyard, and just about everywhere. The Qigong therapies introduced in this book are characterized by easy and practical learning and practice. One can master them even without the instruction of a teacher. Qigong therapies introduced in this book are suitable for all Qigong enthusiasts who wish to be face of diseases, and enjoy a healthy body and a long life.

Contents

Chapter One   Introduction to Qigong   1
  What Is Qigong   1
  The Effects of Qigong   1
  The Essentials of Qigong Practice   2
  Matters Needing Attention   3
  Correcting Deviations from the Path of Qigong   4
Chapter Two   Practical Qigong for Home Health Care   6
  Quiescent Sitting Health Cultivation Exercise   6
  Relaxed and Quiescent Recumbent Exercise   9
  Standing Straight Like a Stake Cultivation Exercise   10
  Morning Walking Exercise   15
  Health Cultivation Massage   16
  Ear Massage to Strengthen Health   18
  Longevity Exercise   20
  Eight Pieces of Brocade Exercise   27
  Sinew-transfroming Exercise   41
  The Buddha's Guardians' Exercise   51
  The Five Animals Frolic   57
  Harmonization Exercise   62
  Taiji Qigong   66
Chapter Three   Qigong Therapy for Some Common Diseases and Serious Diseases   84
  The Common Cold   84
  Neurasthenia   85
  Insomnia   88
  Chronic Bronchitis and Emphysema   89
  Tuberculosis   92
  Bronchial Asthma   93
  Pneumosilicosis   94
  Bronchiectasic Disease   95
  Pneumothorax   96
  Virus Pneumonia   97
  Chronic Gastritis   98
  Gastric and Duodenal Ulcer   99
  Gastroptosia   101
  Volvulus of Stomach   102
  Chronic Hepatitis   103
  Cirrhosis   104
  Cholelithiasis   106
  Intestinal Adhesion   108
  Diarrhea   109
  Constipation   110

Proctoptosis 111
Hemorrhoids 112
Hypotension 114
Hypertension 115
Cerebral Arteriosclerosis 117
Apoplexy Sequelae 118
Coronary Heart Disease 120
Chronic Rheumatic Heart Disease 122
Congestive Heart Failure 124
Chronic Myocarditis 126
Primary Thrombocytopenic Purpura 127
Diaphragm Convulsion 127
Acromelic Arteriospasm 128
Hysteria 129
Facial Nerve Paralysis 130
Rheumatoid Arthritis 131
Cervical Spondylopathy 133
Stiff Neck 135
Scapulohumeral Periarthritis 136
Tennis Elbow 137
Myotenositis of Common Extensor Muscle of the Fingers 138
Prolapse of Lumbar Intervertebral Disc 139
Acute Lumbar Sprain 143
Lumbar Muscle Strain 144
Sciatica 147
Osteophyte 149
Angitis 150
Peripheral Neuritis 151
Chronic Nephritis 152
Sexual Impotence 153
Diabetes Mellitus 154
Prostatomegaly 156
Varicocele 157
Alopecia Areata 158
Vitiligo 159
Chronic Pelvic Inflammation 160
Metroptosis 161
Menopausal Syndrome 162
Dysmenorrhea 162
Menstrual Disorder 163
Dysfunctional Uterine Bleeding 165
Myopia 166
Senile Cataracts 167
Glaucoma 169
Electric Ophthalmia 170

Meniere's Syndrome 171
Laryngopharyngitis 171
Chronic Rhinopathy 172
Chronic Tympanitis 173

Chapter Four   The Accessory Therapeutic Method of Qigong for Carcinosis 175
Nasopharyngeal Carcinoma 175
Pulmonary Carcinoma 177
Esophagus Carcinoma 178
Stomach Carcinoma 180
Hepatic Carcinoma 181
Breast Cancer 182
Cervical Carcinoma 183
Malignant Lymphoma 184
Osteosarcoma 184

Chapter Five   Jingluo and Qigong Point Massage 186
The Distribution of *Jingluo* and Its Functions 186
The Commonly Used Qigong Point Massage 193

Chapter Six   Qigong Massage for Natural Beauty 217
Using Qigong to Make the Face More Beautiful 217
Using Qigong to Make the Neck More Beautiful 220
Exercises for Female Beauty 221
Slimming for Females 223
Body-shaping Exercises 225
Eliminating Fat in the Waist 229
Correction of Humpback 230
Elimination of Double Chins 231
Exercises for Puerperal Restoration 233

Chapter One
INTRODUCTION TO QIGONG

Qigong is a bright pearl in the treasure-house of Chinese medical science. In China it has been a traditional way of maintaining good health for thousands of years, and it is renowned for its magical effect.

WHAT IS QIGONG

Lao Zi, the founder of Daoism who lived during the Spring and Autumn Period (770-476BC), said of *qi*: "in a trance, there is appearance and substance; in gentle and meditation, there is spirit which is truthfulness and has a faith in." In this way, therefore, *qi* is a moving, etherial energy that includes material substance, potential ability, and feedback information. That is *qi*, or rather *zhen qi* (true vital energy), is one's entire life energy; it is the life force which we draw upon in all of our activities. When the *zhen qi* is no more, life ends. The "gong" of Qigong, in the sense of "practice," resonates with its meaning in the compounds *gongdi* (foundation), *gongli* (physical strength), and *gongfu* (or kungfu, literally meaning "power and capability"). Qigong can raise resistance to illness and aid the development of a strong constitution. Through self-control and concentration Qigong can cure disease and prolong life by tapping the potential energy and mobilizing it to maintain life.

THE EFFECTS OF QIGONG

According to modern scientific research in Qigong, it has been shown to have a certain regulating function on the nervous system, respiratory system, digestive system, circulatory system and internal secretion system. Qigong also can promote the balance of yin (negative) and yang (positive) and so maintain the internal stability of the body. It can also help recover one's youthful vigour.

Generally speaking, upon practising Qigong for a period of time some special effects occur, which can be divided into normal and abnormal effects. The following are normal effects:

1. You experience a general ease, your limbs tingle and you sweat a little.

2. The peristalsis of the stomach and intestines increases, which assists regulation of the digestive system.

3. A lessening of both mental and physical fatigue with an improvement in the quality of sleep and appetite.

4. A tickling sensation in the skin which is a sign of improved blood circulation.

5. Muscles twitch and joints pop; this is a sign of an invigorated bodily *zhen qi* (true vital energy or true *qi*).

6. A feeling of tranquillity, comfort and vigour; these are the joyous benefits of mastering the practice. Not everyone experiences these effects, however, so suppress the urge to pursue any one of the above exclusively. Let things take their natural course.

The following are abnormal effects:

1. Increased heart beat and breathlessness. A result of uptightness and unnatural breathing, this can be corrected by relaxing the body.

2. Dry mouth and tickles in the throat. These are caused by breathing with the mouth open or closed tightly. Drink a little warm boiled water before practising and let the tongue lap the roof of the mouth with the mouth half closed.

3. Abdominal distension, with *qi* traveling from the abdomen up into the chest. This is caused by over-concentration and unnatural breathing. It can be solved by relaxing the concentration and breathing naturally.

4. Mental confusion and a dazed feeling. This too can be corrected by relaxing mental concentration and breathing naturally.

5. Headaches and insomnia are also caused by over concentration and being too nervous while practising. It is necessary to relax, lighten the concentration and breathe deeply.

THE ESSENTIALS OF QIGONG PRACTICE

Qigong is an exercise method which is used to regulate the practitioner's bodily functions through introspective action. The positive effects of Qigong build up gradually, level by level with regular and patient practice. Thus, the prescribed sequence of steps must be held to. The following words should be kept in mind: Be full of confidence, be resolute, keep with and work hard at the exercises, and attempt to grasp the essentials of Qigong.

What, then, are the essentials of practising Qigong? There are three: one should both "have" and "not have" concentration. Concretely speaking, this means three dos and three don'ts.

Three dos: Do combine the feeling of "getting together" and "breaking up";

Do perform what is apparently right but actually wrong;

Do achieve a state of letting go of thoughts.

Three don'ts: Don't practise with strain;

Don't become excited;

Don't harbour a goal.

Since concentration of mind is based on the regular movement of *qi*, which is transmitted by the concentration of mind, the body can become relaxed and the mind can reach motionlessness (a high stage of Qigong) by following the rule, "concentration of mind goes with *qi*."

Breathing—should be natural, light, even, long, and soft—as silkworms spin silk into an unbroken filament. The beginner should be sure to breathe naturally and slowly; people who suffer from a disease should breathe from the abdomen. There are two kinds of abdominal respirations: bloating the abdomen when inhaling and pulling in the abdomen on exhaling, or pulling in the abdomen when inhaling and bloating it on exhaling. The advantage of abdominal respiration is the clearing up of harmful gas and the massaging of the stomach, intestines, liver and gall. During this process, digestive functions and some other organs' functions are regulated, and some diseases may receive incidental treatment.

Posture—that is to say, regulation of the body's carriage, including the head, neck, waist, limbs, fingers and internal organs. For exmaple, Wo Gong (Relaxed and Quiescent Lying Exercise) regulates the limbs and internal organs. Zhan Gong (Standing Exercise) regulates the head and waist. Zuo Gong (Quiescent Sitting Exercise) regulates the head, waist, neck, legs and hands. The basic principle of correct posture is to find the position in which the body is the most comfortable.

MATTERS NEEDING ATTENTION

Qigong is a science. In order to avoid side effects, an aspiring Qigong practitioner should not regard himself or herself as infallible. Allow yourself to learn. In particular, these following matters need attention:

1. Keep your mind in a cheerful frame while exercising, putting behind any vexing matter or thoughts that make you excited. Otherwise, stop exercising and take a rest, go for a walk or do something else until you quiet down and feel at ease.

2. Keep your body still. A half hour before practising Qigong, you should stop strenuous activities, both physical and mental, in order to relax the muscles and mind.

3. Your stomach should be neither too full nor too empty at practice time. Eating very cold or hot and spicy foods before practice is not allowed.

4. Practise warm-down exercise. Qigong masters often say: "If one doesn't practise warm-down exercise, it would be better not to practise Qigong at all." Warm-down exercise is a very important step in the process of practising Qigong, and it links with the process. First, one should mentally prepare for the warm-down Qigong, reciting three times silently: "I am going to conclude my exercise." At the same time, keep your feelings stable and cheerful. Don't open your eyes impatiently or stop your exercise abruptly, and don't stand facing the wind.

CORRECTING DEVIATIONS FROM THE PATH OF QIGONG

Generally speaking, if you follow the prescribed order of the exercises and pay attention to the matters described above, no deviations will occur. If there is a deviation, you can correct it with one of the following methods:

1. Relaxed and Quiescent Method

Lie down or sit on a chair peacefully and comfortably, cross the hands placing the two tiger's mouths (part of the hand between the thumb and the forefinger) against each other and then put them across the lower belly. Breathe out once gently, then, using *yinian* (concentration of the mind), transmit *qi* from the head downward gradually, while reciting "relax... relax... relax..." quietly to yourself. Do this twice a day, each time about 15 to 20 minutes. After a time of practising this exercise, suffering will be alleviated and Qigong will once again be able to be performed with a relaxed and even-tempered feeling.

2. Transmit *Qi* with Movement Method

1) Standing with feet apart at a distance of a little more than the width of the shoulders. While slowly taking in a breath, move the arms from the sides in an arc forward slowly and evenly, bringing the hands together at the level of the larynx as you reach the end of the inhale. Then exhale, moving the hands with the palms face down, slowly down along the middle line of the torso. At the same time, think to transmit *qi* downward, while bending the knees to half squat. Your hands should reach your lower abdomen just as the exhale ends and then separate them. Then repeat the inhale motions, straightening the legs. Repeat the above movements several times.

2) Standing naturally, extend the arms forward as if carrying a tree; when you breathe in, move the arms in an arc outward; when you breathe out, arms draw in, bend the knees in half squat. The movement of the upper and lower limbs should be coordinated. Rise up slowly to a natural standing position and repeat the sequence.

Through this exercise, the *qi* goes up and down in a regular cycle to correct any imbalance in the *qi*'s function.

3. Method of the Three Lines Penetrating *Qi*

When you breathe in, concentrate your mind on Dantian (in the lower abdomen); when you breathe out, release harmful gases following the three lines described below:

1) Release the harmful gases following an imaginary line drawn from the face to the chest, from the chest to the abdomen, from the abdomen to the inner sides of the legs and from the legs inside to the Yongquan point.

2) Release the harmful gases from the head to the shoulders, from the shoulders to the arms, from the arms to the fingertips.

3) From the crown of the head down tips to the back, to the buttocks, to the

outer side of the legs and down to the backside of the legs to the toes releasing the harmful gases.

4. Six-word Respiration Exercise

Standing naturally and hands hanging loosely, relax yourself. As you breathe in, concentrate your mind on Dantian; as you breathe out, recite these following six words silently:

Xu—slowly breathe out the liver's *qi*.

He—breathe out with the mouth open the heart's *qi*.

Hu—exhale the spleen's *qi*.

Si—breathe out with the mouth half opened the lung's *qi*.

Chui—blow out the kidney's *qi*.

Xi—breathe out with the mouth lightly closed the Sanjiao Jing's *qi*.

5. Point Massage

Personally or have someone else use the palm, thumb or middle finger to massage Taiyang, Dazhui, Shanzhong, Yongquan, Qihai and other points to stimulate the channels and blood vessels rotating in only one direction.

6. Patting the Internal Organs

Standing naturally, lightly pat the body with the palms, or have another person lightly pat, along one of the body's lines, in order to shake loose the blood circulation and *qi*, stimulate the channels, and regulate the organ's function.

7. Free-walking Exercise

Should you become utterly confused and disconcerted during practice, stop for a few days and do some free walking, turning your attention to the scenery around you in order to relax yourself.

8. Regulation Exercise

See Chapter Two for details.

9. Longevity Exercise

See Chapter Two for details.

When you experience a deviation caused by incorrect practice of Qigong which you cannot solve by yourself, please consult with a Qigong master or Qigong doctor at a Qigong hospital. There the deviation can be corrected and treated.

Chapter Two
PRACTICAL QIGONG FOR HOME HEALTH CARE

The purposes of home care Qigong are the curing of disease and prolonging of life. Though there are many kinds of home care Qigong, the main division of techniques comes between *neigong* (internal exercise) and *waigong* (external exercise). Those practised mainly in a quiescent state are called internal exercise or quiescent exercise, characterized by concentrating attention on Dantian (the elixir field) in concert with inhalation, exhalation and holding of breath in order to stimulate *qi* (vital energy) and blood and to build up the five internal organs, such as Quiescent Sitting Health Cultivation Exercise, Relaxed and Quiescent Exercise, Standing-Straight Like a Stake Exercise, Taiji Qigong. Those practised mainly with mobile exercise are called external exercise, characterized by "external mobility and internal quiescence, seeking quiescence within mobility," such as Eight-Pieces-of-Brocade Exercise, Sinew-Transforming Exercise, the Five Animals Frolic.

Internal exercise and external exercise can be practised either singly or in concert. For people with a weak constitution, internal exercise can be done alone at the start, with external exercise being added after the constitution becomes stronger. Because there are many kinds of Qigong, one should select appropriate kind or kinds according to individual characteristics and capabilities. As for the purpose of health care only, one or two kinds of Qigong can be exercised. However, according to the practical experience of exercisers, it is most suitable to combine internal exercise with external exercise. Thus, both mobility and quiescence are included, externality and internality are integrated together, and twice the result will be obtained with half the effort.

QUIESCENT SITTING HEALTH CULTIVATION EXERCISE
(Jing Zuo Yang Sheng Gong)

Sitting quiescently is an effective measure for adjusting cerebral function. Ancient Chinese called it "the method of cultivation through sitting quiescently" or "the quiescent method." "Quiescence" is practised on the basis of relaxing and being at ease. It can soothe the cerebrum, make one to be even tempered and good-humoured, give the nerve center an opportunity for rest and reorganization. Sitting quiescently for half hour periods will have therapeutic effect for diseases of the nervous, circulatory and digestive systems and will also achieve unique results for exploiting intelligence and putting off the aging process.

1. Postures

1) Sitting style: sit upright with eyes and mouth closed lightly. Let the head and neck be straight and hang the head slightly forward. Pull in the chest a little. Put the feet horizontally at a distance of about the width of the shoulders. Lower the shoulders, bend the elbows slightly, put the hands on the thighs naturally with the palms facing down, and relax the whole body. (Figs.1-1, 2)

2) Crossed limbs style: the posture is the same as that of the sitting style with the exception of crossing both hands on the lower part of the underbelly. For a male, the left hand is placed against the body and the thumb is put at the third joint of the ring finger, while the four fingers of the right hand are placed externally with the thumb inserted into the center of the palm of the left hand. The ankles of both feet are crossed with the left foot behind the right one. The angle between thigh and shank is 60 degrees. For female persons, the positions of hands and feet are opposite. (Fig. 2)

2. Two Kinds of Respiration

1) The first kind: inhale—hold breath—exhale, reciting silently "I—want quiescent—sitting" (breaking the phrase into three, one for each action). The procedure is: Close the mouth, touching the upper palate with the tip of tongue. Recite silently the word "I" while inhaling through the nostrils, recite "want quiescent" silently without moving the mouth and tongue, with the breath held, then drop the tongue and recite silently the word "sitting" while exhaling through

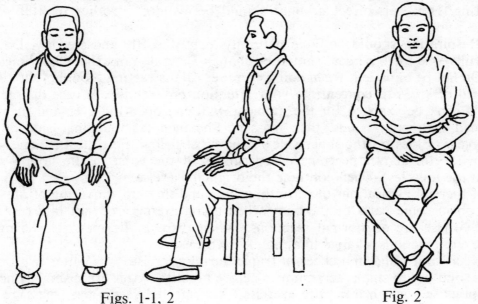

Figs. 1-1, 2   Fig. 2

the mouth. Repeat this for 30 minutes or so.

2) The second kind: inhale—exhale—hold breath, reciting silently "I—want —quiescent sitting" (again, in three parts). The procedure is: recite silently the word "I" while inhaling through the nostrils, read "want" while exhaling throgh the mouth and dropping the tongue, recite "quiecent sitting" while holding the breath with the closed mouth and the tongue touching the upper palate. Repeat this for about 30 minutes.

3. Concentration of Mind

1) When practising the first method of respiration, the mind should be concentrated on the Shanzhong point (at the centre of the line drawn between the nipples) of the middle Dantian, or on the Baihui point (at the centre of the line drawn between the ears). One of these two acupoints can be chosen. "Concentration" means that the attention should be concentrated on that position from the beginning till the end of practising the exercise. In addition, inflate the lower belly slightly during inhalation in order to send the clear *qi* to penetrate the Dantian below the navel. Draw in the lower belly when exhaling.

2) When the second method is performed, the mind should be concentrated on the Guanyuan point (at the distance of four times the diameter of a finger below the navel). Inflate the lower part of the abdomen below the navel during inhalation, take it in when exhaling and holding the breath, trying your best to keep this condition for the sake of allowing the remaining *qi* to be brought into the lower Dantian.

4. Matters Needing Attention

1) The exercise area should not be too bright and the air should be freely circulating. However, direct draught should be avoided in order to keep from catching cold.

2) Respiration should be done naturally, gently, softly and steadily. Do not inhale fully—80 to 90 percent should be enough—and do not exhale too violently.

3) Do not be impatient when doing exercise. All distracting thoughts should be gotten rid of so as to concentrate your attention on exercise. In case distracting thoughts can't be expelled for the moment, you can open the eyes and massage your head with both hands, then massage Shenmen (at the ulnar side of the transverse wrinkles on the inner side of the wrist below the pisiform bone) and Neiguan (2 cun above the transverse wrinkles of the wrist in the hollow area between the muscles). Then contiune the original exercise.

4) If there are sensations of warmth, aching and tingling, quivering of muscles and so on in some parts of the body when doing exercise, do not interrupt the exercise—these are all normal reactions. When there is dizziness, fluttering or other severe reactions, change to a mobile exercise.

5) Keep your mind in a cheerful frame during exercise. It is better to stop all activities and not to smoke ten minutes before practice. After exercising, stand up softly, practise some health care exercise, do some light activities, massage the

limbs, and avoid being in a draught for a while.

RELAXED AND QUIESCENT RECUMBENT EXERCISE
(Song Jing Wo Gong)

Proper relaxation of the body, natural breathing, and a peaceful mind are necessary for practising this exercise. It is suitable to the elderly and weak people, neurastheniacs, and people who have no time to exercise at daytime due to a busy work schedule. Practise it before sleep every night, during the night if sleeping unsoundly, and after awakening in the morning. Relaxed and Quiescent Recumbent Exercise quickly inhibit the cerebral cortex and regulate the function of the autonomic nerve, promote the passing of *qi* and help unblock blood circulation, and thus reinforce the physique and cure disease.

1. Postures

1) Flat-back lying style: Lie supine on a pillow of moderate height. Lightly close eyes and mouth. Stretch both arms straight naturally and, with the hands bent a little, put them at the sides of the body. Stretch both legs straight naturally with feet apart slightly and relax the whole body. (Fig. 3)

2) Slanted back lying style: Lie supine on a pillow put on a folded quilt. The body above the waist should be lying on the quilt, forming an incline plane. The posture is the same as above. (Fig. 4)

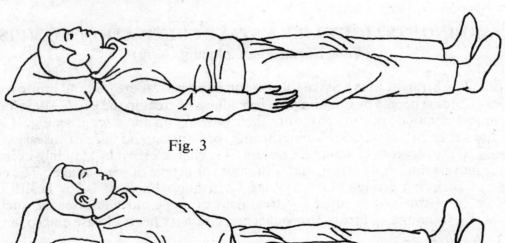

Fig. 3

Fig. 4

3) Side-lying style: Lie on left or right side with a pillow of moderate height. When you lie on the right side, stretch the right leg straight, laying the left leg on the right one and slightly bending the left knee. Bend the right forearm upward and put the right hand near the head with the fingers slightly straightened near the right side of face. Put the left arm on the left side of the body and bend the fingers slightly on the outer side of the left leg. Lightly close eyes and mouth. Relax the whole body. (Fig. 5)

4) Back-lying and ball holding style: Bend both knees, stretch both hands upward and suspend them in midair with the palms down. Point the fingers of each hand towards those of the other, with a distance of 30 cm between them, as if holding a ball. Imagine that you are holding a ball. You will experience a tingling sensation, and a warmth or distension in the center of palms, even the whole body. When the arms are tired lay them down slowly and let the elbows fall on the bed. (Figs. 6-1, 2)

Respiration: Same as that of Quiescent Sitting Health Cultivation Exercise except that the words read silently during respiration are changed to "I—want quiescent—lying" or "I—want—quiescent lying" (depending on the beathing style)

2. Matters Needing Attention

Besides the matters noted in the section on Quiescent Sitting Health Cultivation Exercise, it is also to be noted that the Relaxed and Quiescent Recumbent Exercise can easily lead to sleep. One should persist with the exercise for at least half an hour before going to sleep.

STANDING STRAIGHT LIKE A STAKE CULTIVATION EXERCISE
(Yang Sheng Zhan Zhuang Gong)

Standing Straight Like a Stake Cultivation Exercise was created and improved by ancient Chinese people by imitating the rootedness of trees in the earth—developing a firm and immobile posture to ensure their growing up and strengthening. It is an exercise for health care, body strengthening, prevention and cure of diseases, and belongs to the category of internal exercise. It is characterised by standing exercise, simple movements, rapid effect, and is suitable for people of various ages. The chief usage of Standing Straight Like a Stake Cultivation Exercise is for health care —however, it can also be used for treatment of some chronic diseases, such as headaches, insomnia, neurosis, stomachaches, coronary heart disease and so on.

1. Postures

1) Natural standing style: separate the feet in the width of the shoulders parallel. Keep the head upright and pull in the chest slightly. Slightly bend the knees. Put the hands on the lower belly with the left hand inside and the right one outside, palms facing inwards. Eyes look horizontally or downwards. (Fig. 7)

2) Cupping standing style: Standing with the feet apart as above, let the eyes

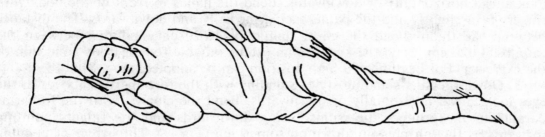

Fig. 5

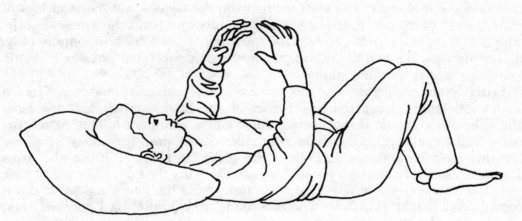

Fig. 6-1

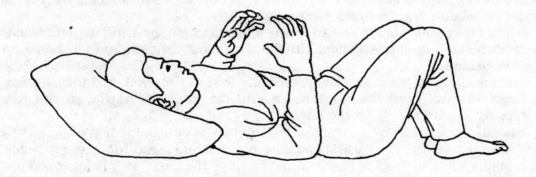

Fig. 6-2

look ahead horizontally or downwards. Bend the hands in front of the body with fingers bent slightly and the palms facing medially and downwards. The distance between the thumbs and the chest should be 16-20 cm, and that between the thumbs, 13-20 cm. Bend the knees to an extent suitable for the body condition of the exerciser. For beginners, a high position can be adopted. (Fig. 8)

3) Down-pressing standing style: Standing with the feet apart as above, let the eyes look ahead horizontally or downwards. Bend the elbows, with the forearms parallel to the ground, the palms facing downwards and the fingers pointing forwards as though pressing down on something (Fig. 9). The extent of bending of the knees can be different according to the body condition of the exerciser.

4) Hands-on-a-chair standing style: Put a chair in front of you. Stand with the feet a shoulder width apart. The distance between the tiptoes and the hind legs of the chair should be 30 cm. Pull in the chest slightly and bend the knees slightly. Rest the hands on the top of the back of the chair. Eyes look horizontally (Fig. 10) or downwards. This style is suitable for people who are physically weak, hemiplegia or unable to stand stably.

5) Mixed standing style: a. Arms lowered and relaxed. Stand with feet a shoulder width apart. Keep the upper part of the body straight and the head upright. The eyes should look horizontally. Close the mouth and lower the shoulders. Hang the arms naturally at your sides. Relax the whole body.

b. Arms stretching forward. Follow the previous posture. Raise the arms simultaneously and stretch them forward without moving the body. The palms face downward and fingers forward. At the same time, bend the knees and squat down to a comfortable height. For those who have done the exercise for a long time and those with good health, squat down as low as possible, or until the thighs are parallel to the ground, without moving the knees forward beyond the tiptoes.

c. Then turn the hands with the palms facing each other without moving the head, neck, chest, abdomen, legs and feet.

d. Slowly draw the hands to the front of the chest with palms facing backwards and let the middle fingers touch each other lightly.

e. Then move the hands outward slowly and straighten the arms, with the hands on the same level as the shoulders. Stretch the fingers straight and let the palms face the ground.

f. Bring the arms together slowly, medially toward the chest, and then straighten them forward. Press the hands down with the palms facing the ground to a distance of 33 cm apart from the knees.

Each of the above movements require 5 minutes. After completion of practising them in order, restore the natural standing position and stand for 2 to 3 minutes. Then inhale while lifting the hands to the front of the chest with palms up. Turn the hands and press them down during exhalation. Bend the knees. These movements should be repeated 3 to 5 times.

For beginners and those with weak constitution, the natural standing style is better to be adopted and the mixed standing one can be exercised after the constitution becomes stronger.

2. Respiration

1) Natural respiration method: Beginners can use their own ordinary natural respiration.

2) Abdominal respiration method: This can be used by exercisers who have practised for a long period. The breath should be slow, even, light and deep. Raise the chest and inflate the lower belly during inhalation and draw back the lower belly for expelling the gas as much as possible during exhalation.

3. Concentration of Mind

1) Common method: This method is suitable for beginners. Attention should be paid only to the posture and the regulation of respiration. One can think of something happy and relaxed.

2) Concentration of mind on Dantian method: When inhalation, think of the natural *qi* being transmitted into Dantian, then hold the breath and concentrate the mind on Dantian. After that, guide down the *qi* of Dantian to the Huiyin point

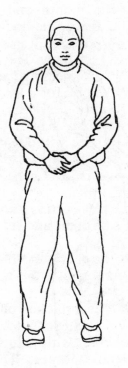

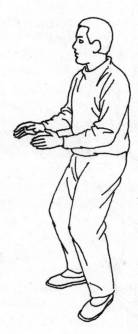

Fig. 7   Fig. 8

(between external genital organ and anus), then upwards to Mingmen on the waist and let it penetrate to the Shenshu points in both sides. Continue to hold the breath and transmit the *qi* from Shenshu downwards along the back of both legs (the Pangguang Jing channels) to Yongquan in the sole, then from Yongquan upwards along the inner side of both legs (the Shen Jing channels) back to Dantian again. Exhale the harmful gas slowly through the mouth. Repeat the above movements. Breathing should be done lightly, long, softly, slowly, gently and naturally.

4. Conclusion of Exercise

No matter what style of the standing cultivation exercise is practised, the legs should be straightened slowly at the end of the exercise and both hands lifted up to the front of chest with the palms facing up and the tips of fingers opposing as a breath is deeply inhaled. Then turn the palms downward and drop the hands from the chest and exhale the gas gradually. Repeat 3 to 5 times successively, then end the exercise.

After the ending of the exercise rub the palms together until they become warm, then gently rub both checks with the palms and pat and massage the head, neck and finally the four limbs by hands. Relax the whole body.

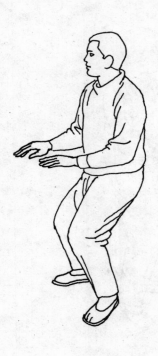

Fig. 9

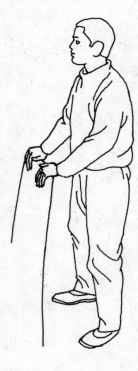

Fig. 10

5. Matters Needing Attention

1) For beginners, the elderly or patients with hypertension and cardiovascular diseases, the natural standing style, natural respiration and common method should be practised.

2) During exercise, accurate and comfortable postures are required. The neck should not be rigid and the whole body should be relaxed, with a happy and easy frame of mind. When one is hungry, having eaten too much, or overworked, it is not suitable to do the exercise. The best time is in the early morning and before going to bed at night.

3) Avoid being caught in a draft or catching cold during exercise. The room should be kept clean and the air fresh when practising inside.

4) If there are sensations of warmth, soreness, numbness or trembling of muscles in some part of the body, quivering slightly at the tips of fingers or in the legs during exercise, do not worry, for all these are normal phenomena. However, do not seek these sensations deliberately. Sensations of warmth in one shoulder and coldness in the other, or even coldness on one side of the body and warmth on the other, are due to imbalance of yin and yang, stimulation of the vital energy and blood, and obstruction of channels and collaterals. The exercise should be continued, as all of these symptoms will disappear as soon as the channels and collaterals are cleared and the harmony between yin and yang reestablished.

5) When the exerciser feels cold throughout the body or shivers during practice, the exercise should be stopped at once. Do self-massage or wash the hands and face with hot water and drink hot tea to restore the normal state. However, exercise should not be done again till next day. If the above-mentioned symptoms appear more than three times successively, other exercise methods should be practised.

6) If there are symptoms of asthenia, sweating and dizziness during practice of the concentration of mind on Dantian method, it is due to overlong holding of the breath; hence the latter should be stopped and the common method should be adopted. When practising on the next day, one should concentrate on mastering the proper holding of the breath. The principle of proceeding in an orderly way, step by step, should be followed in doing the exercise. Do not act with undue haste.

MORNING WALKING EXERCISE
(Chen Bu Gong)

The ancient Chinese people said "Wake up as soon as the cock crows to stroll in the courtyard and ease the mind. This is the so-called way of cultivation." To walk in the morning and inhale fresh air is a kind of traditional health care method of the Chinese people. It is appropriate especially for old people. A better effect can be had when Qigong exercises are practised in addition.

1. Exercise Method

1) Rest a while before strolling in the morning. With eyes looking forward on a horizontal line towards a distant object, stare for a moment. Be in a good mood and have ease of spirit. After "spitting" qi out of mouth three times, inhale deeply through the nostrils. At the first inhale swallow the qi down into the chest as if swallowing food. Think the qi is sent to Dantian in the belly during the second inhale. During the third inhale, transmit it down to the feet. Then keep quiet for a while.

2) Stand straight before strolling, with neck straight, chin relaxed towards the chest and shoulders lowered. Then inhale successively three times. On each inhale, contract the belly inwards, lifting the anus and testes at the same time, then exhale strenuouslly through the mouth. After the whole body is relaxed, step forward to begin the stroll. Be leisurely, carefree, happy and relaxed during walking. Inhale through nose once at each step, counting silently. Inhale 8 times for 8 steps. Inhalation should be done through the nose violently, suddenly and deeply, with jingling sounds. Stop moving forward at the ninth step and inhale through the nose. Continue strolling after a rest. It is very advantageous to perform this exercise repeatedly in this way and persist in doing it every morning. For old and weak people, the natural respiration method is to be used chiefly, and concentration on breathing can be gradually increased.

HEALTH CULTIVATION MASSAGE
(An Mo Yang Sheng Fa)

Health Cultivation Massage belongs to the mobile cultivation methods of Qigong exercises. It is characterized by "cultivation by movements" that are simple and easily done. In the Ming Dynasty (1368-1644) this method was popularized among the Chinese people. It is good for health care, body strengthening and prolonging life if exercised frequently and persistently.

1. Exercise Method

1) Combing the hair. The acuity of vision can be improved and the pathogenic wind be expelled by combing one's hair frequently. The method is to comb hair softly in the morning, and repeat this ten times a day.

2) Dry-washing the face. Pathogenic factors can be eliminated through frequent face washing—and an added effect is that no wrinkles will appear on the shiny face. Method: rub the hands until they are warm, then put them on the nose and scrub upward along both sides of the nose mainly with the middle fingers. After the fingers reach the forehead, separate them and slide them down lightly along both sides of the forehead. Repeat the movement 30 times.

3) Moving the eyeballs. Cataracts and nebula can be eliminated and the near

and far-sightedness corrected through exercising the eyeballs frequently. Method: rotate the eyeballs first from left to right then from right to left. These movements should be done slowly. After rotating in both directions 14 times each, close the eyes tightly for a while and then open them wide suddenly and "wield" the eyesight.

4) Knocking the ears. Dizziness and tinnitus can be prevented and cured by frequent knocking of the ears. Method: Cover the ear canals with both palms and press the index fingers upon the middle fingers. Knock the back part of the skull lightly with the index fingers 24 times.

5) Tapping the teeth. Teeth tapping can improve the roots of the teeth without pain. Method: Chomp the upper and lower teeth together as though chewing food. Tap in both upward and downward directions 24 times each.

6) Licking the palate. The ancient Chinese regarded the saliva as the treasure of the human body and called it "the golden juice" and "jade wine." Licking the palate with the tongue can stimulate saliva production. Method: Lick between the lips and teeth with the tip of tongue, moving from left to right, then from right to left. Repeat 30 times each.

7) Swallowing the saliva. The ancient Chinese considered swallowing the saliva as a way to irrigate the "five visceral organs" and "six bowels" and moisten the limbs, joints and body hair. Method: Lick the upper palate with the tongue and gargle with the resulting saliva 36 times. Then swallow lightly the saliva in three mouthfuls.

8) Inflating the chest. By doing this, stagnated food can be moved away and fullness in the chest and diaphragm can be eliminated. Method: Hold the breath and inflate the chest and the belly. When the maximal inflating has been gained, raise the head, open the mouth and puff out the harmful gas. It is appropriate to repeat this 5 to 7 times.

9) Rubbing the belly. Rubbing the belly can soothe the mind and move along stagnated food. Method: Rub the palms together until they are warm, then lay them together on the bare belly directly or on an unlined garment. Rub the belly clockwise with the center of the palm moving circularly around the navel. Making small, medium-sized and large circles twelve times each.

10) Contracting the sphincter. The ancient Chinese called this lifting the passway of rice. This exercise can make the yang (positive) qi rise up. Method: Inhale with some strength and contract the muscles of the anus and the perineum. Hold this for a while, then relax the muscles and exhale. Exercise this 5 to 7 times.

11) Rocking the limbs. This exercise can limber up the joints of the four limbs. Method: Grasp both shoulders with the hands firmly. Turn the left shoulder to the front first, then turn the right one forward, as if turning a winch. Turn the shoulders in both directions 24 times each, then sit stably. Lift the left foot and stretch its tip upward slowly. When the left leg is almost stretched straight, kick the left heel out suddenly. Repeat the movements five times. After that, change

the right foot to do the same movement.

12) Rubbing the foot's arch. The ancient Chinese called this "Rubbing Yongquan." Yongquan is an acupuncture point at the fore part of the underside of the foot arch (one third of the down the sole from the toes). Rubbing this point can reinforce the kidney, warm the foot, facilitate the interconnection between the heart and the kidney, and depress the deficiency fire, thus helping the exerciser to go to sleep. Rub the left foot first and then the right one. Repeat the movement 50 to 100 times for each foot.

13) Dry bath. Dry bathing can smooth the circulation of *qi* and blood and make the skin lustrous and smooth. Method: Rub the hands until they are warm, then rub the body. The order of rubbing is generally from the Baihui to the face, passing over the left and right shoulders, both arms, the chest and the belly then along the sides of the torso to the waist, and at last the legs.

14) Relaxing the muscles and tendons. The ancient Chinese considered this exercise capable of relaxing the muscles and tendons and activating the flow of *qi* and blood in the channels and collaterals. Method: Sitting on the bed with both legs stretched straight. Lower the head forward and pull the foot arch with both hands simultaneously twelve times. Clap the thighs and shanks several times during the intervals.

For the above-mentioned methods of cultivation, it is better to perform the exercise of combing the hair in the early morning, the exercises of washing face and relaxing muscles and tendons after waking up, the exercise of rubbing Yongquan after washing the feet and before going to sleep. Practise the other ten exercises twice daily. They can be exercised as a group or a part of them can be selected to practise.

EAR MASSAGE TO STRENGTHEN HEALTH
(Rou Er Jian Shen Fa)

The ear is a microcosm of the human body—even its form looks like a fetus suspended upside down within the belly of its mother. It was said in ancient Chinese medical books that there is a close relationship between the ear auricle and the channels and collaterals. Clinical observation reveals that the physiological and pathological status of internal organs is approximately reflected at the corresponding locations of the auricle. Hence, rubbing the auricles frequently can stimulate the channels and collaterals, regulate the excitatory and inhibitory processes of the nerves, enhance metabolic function, and promote blood circulation. Therefore, it is very good for the prevention and cure of diseases and strengthening of the constitution. The exercise is simple, safe but not time-consuming, and is especially suitable for the elderly.

1.Exercise Method

1) Rubbing the auricle with the fingers. With the thumb and the index finger opposing each other, put them on the front and back sides of the auricle. Rub both auricles beginning from the upper end down to the earlobe in a spiral way. Repeat several times. There are altogether three bands on the auricle. Rub from the helix to the middle zone, then from middle zone to the ear root zone several times until the auricle becomes warm. (Fig. 11)

2) Kneading the auricular points. After the auricle has been rubbed warm, knead the acupoints on the auricle related to the exerciser's diseases with the nail of the index finger 2 to 3 times until there is slight pain. When the exact points are not known by the exerciser, all the concave and convex parts can be kneaded, with some sensitive points being stressed wherever they are found. If the same action as acupuncture is achieved, better effects will be gained. (Fig. 12)

3) Twisting the root of the auricle. Push the pad of the thumb with some strength from Yifeng point behind the earlobe upward to the upper end of the auricle. Then push the index finger from the front upper end downward to the front side of the earlobe. Repeat in this way 5 to 10 times. (Fig. 13-1)

4) Pulling both auricles. Bend the thumbs and the index fingers of both hands, hold the cartilage in the lower part of the ear with the tips of the fingers, pull the auricles laterally until slight pain is felt in the external auditory canal. Then shake and pull the auricles lightly downward and laterally one after another until there is a sensation in the external auditory canal. Generally one can pull many times, even 200 to 300 times, according to individual conditions. (Fig. 13-2)

2. Matters Needing Attention

The massaging should be done softly in the beginning and become heavier gradually until a comfortable sensation is attained. Do the massage once or twice

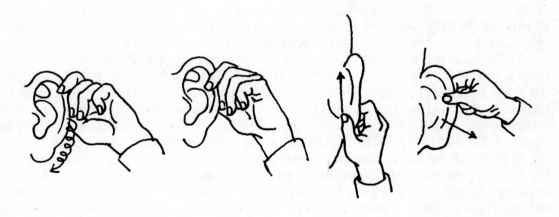

Fig. 11   Fig. 12   Fig. 13-1   Fig. 13-2

a day. If there is frostbite or trauma on the auricle, the exercise should be suspended for prevention of infection.

LONGEVITY EXERCISE
(Chang Shou Gong)

Chang Shou Gong has been popular in the Taihu (Lake Taihu) Region of South China for a long time. It is characterized by integration of mobile and quiescent exercises, convenience for practice both on land or in a boat, providing firmness and gentleness, and all-round positive effects. When it is practised persistently, the diseases may be cured and prolonging of life obtained.

1.Exercise Method

1) The preparatory posture. Calm the mind and concentrate the thoughts, but do not be slack. Let Baihui face the sky. Lower the shoulders and drop elbows. Keep the armpits open, pull in the chest, tense the abdomen, relax the hips, contract the sphincter and bend the knees slightly, standing with the feet a shoulder width apart. Close the mouth and eyes slightly, touch the upper palate with the tip of tongue and breathe naturally. It is generally appropriate to stand in this way for 1 to 5 minutes. This posture is used both at the beginning and end of the exercise.

2) Looking at the moon from the prow of a boat. Stand with feet a shoulder width apart and arms akimbo. Turn the head at first to the upper right with the eyes looking up the sky, and inhale sufficient air. Then, turn the head downward and exhale slowly (Fig. 14). Repeat the movements in this way 10 to 15 times.

3) Intercepting on the waist. Standing with feet a shoulder width apart. Put both hands on the back, with the centre of the back of one hand pressing lightly and accurately on the Shenshu of the same side and the palm of other hand covering accurately the Shenshu point of the other side, and rubbing it upward and downward 30 to 50 rounds. Then rub the opposite side with the palm of that side (Fig. 15). Repeat the movements, alternating 2 to 4 times.

4) Pushing the boat along with the current. Standing with feet a little wider than a shoulder width apart. Put the left hand on the side of the waist and push the right palm to the upper right until the arm is stretched straight. At the same time turn the head to the left with the eyes looking forward and inhale. After that, return to the original position and exhale. Then, do the same movements with the opposite hand (Fig. 16-1). Repeat, alternating 10 to 20 times.

5) Pushing the waves back and forth. Standing in the bow stance with the right leg at the front, push the right arm forward with the palm facing the front while drawing the left arm backward with its palm facing the back, and inhale. Then change the position of both arms and do the same movements, exhaling when changing. Repeat this 10 to 15 times. Then change the position of the legs and do the same movements. Repeat with alternated legs 2 to 4 times (Fig. 16-2).

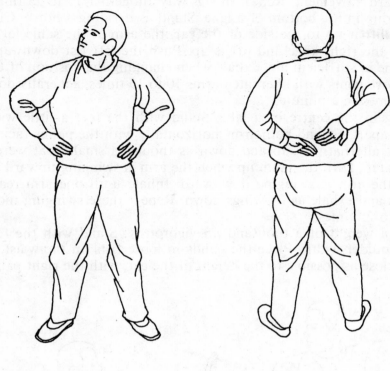

Fig. 14   Fig. 15

6) One-armed general. Stand with feet separated by a little more than a shoulder width. Put the left hand on the side of the waist and stretch straight the right arm to the right horizontally. Make circles with 12 cm in diametre with the right arm, taking the shoulder joint as the axis. Breathe once for each circle. Rotate clockwise and counterclockwise, ten circles each. Then change the position of the arms. Repeat the movements with alternated arms 4 to 6 times.

7) Wave upon waves. Stand with feet separated by a little more than a shoulder width. Extend both arms to the sides horizontally, inhaling at the same time. Then push the arms down the front to the knees, bending the upper part of the body. Touch the hollow of the knee with little fingers (Fig. 17), exhaling at the same time. After exhaling, stand straight with the chest throwing out. Extend both arms to the sides horizontally and look at the sky, inhaling at the same time. Repeat the movements in this way 10 to 20 times.

8) Seething waters up and down. Stand with feet a little wider than a shoulder width apart. Clench both hands loosely and lift them up, but not beyond the level of the ear. Simultaneously rotate the arms forward defining circles 15 cm in diametre. Breathe once for one circle. Inhale during rotating upward while exhale

during down ward movement. Repeat in this way altogether 15 to 25 times.

9) Adventuring in the bottom of a lake. Stand as if riding a horse. Clench the right hand and lift it up to the side of the ear, the arm at the same level as the shoulder. Bend the right knee and lift it up. Push the left fist downward to the right and breathe in sufficient air. Exhale when changing the position of the arms. Repeat these movements with alternated arms 10 to 15 times, generally doing it no more than 10 times in a minute.

10) Rocking in the centre of a lake. Stand with the feet a little wider than shoulder width apart. Extend both arms horizontally with the palms facing down. Swing the arms alternatively up and down as though a small boat were tossing about on the water. Turn the palm up when the arm is swinging upward and turn it down when the arm is swinging downward. Inhale until one arm reaches the maximal height and exhale as it swings down. Repeat these swinging movements in this way 15 to 25 times.

11) Lifting a weight of a thousand *jin* vigorously. Stand with the feet apart more than a shoulder width. Place the hands in loose fists on the waist. Lift the right elbow as close as possible to the height of the ear, with the right palm facing

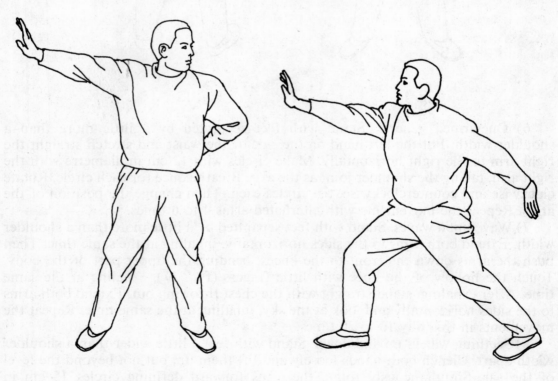

Fig. 16-1   Fig. 16-2

backward. Then lift it higher with strength and at the same time throw out the chest, tense the belly and inhale twice vigourously with sound (Fig. 18). Exhale when lowering the right elbow to the same height as that of the left one. Change the position of the arms and do the same movements. Repeat 15 to 25 times.

12) Going forward by cleaving the waves. Stand with feet a shoulder width apart. Clench both hands and, with the palms facing down, put the fists on the sides of the waist. With the right leg step forward about half a pace, bend the upper part of the body backward slightly. Extend both fists forward horizontally and lean the upper part of the body forward. Throw out the chest, inhale, bend the front leg slightly and stretch the back leg straight. Restore the former position. Then stretch the front leg straight while bending the back leg slightly and exhaling. Repeat these back and forth movements 10 to 20 times. After that, change to the other leg to do the same.

13) Tiger's back and bear's waist. Stand with the feet apart slightly more than a shoulder width. Alternating, touch the back and the waist; the hands should reach the level of the first thoracic vertebra. Throw out the chest and inhale when the right hand is touching the back. Exhale when changing hands. Repeat 15 to 20 times, at a rate of not more than 10 times a minute.

14) Bending legs and moving knees. Stand with the feet apart at a shoulder width. Bend the hips, knees and ankles, covering the knees with both palms. Rotate the palms both clockwise and counterclockwise 15 times each. After that, restore the original posture.

15) Dispelling the waves at left and right sides. Stand with the feet a little wider than a shoulder width apart. Put both palms in front of the chest with their centres facing each other and the fingers pointing up. Push the right hand to the right side as though dispelling the waves, with the palm facing the right until the right arm is stretched horizontal, inhaling at the same time. Restore the right hand to its former place while exhaling. Then do the expelling movement with the left hand to the left side. Repeat this way 15 to 25 times. Essentials: the eyes should be look at the fingers of the moving hand.

16) A dolphin leaping out of water. Stand with the feet apart wider of the shoulders. Let the arms hang naturally at your sides. Begin the exercise by rotating both arms simultaneously to the back, then upward, inhaling at the same time. Jump up once or raise the heel up once when the hands reach their highest point. After that, rotate both arms simultaneously forward, then downward and exhale. Repeat the arms-rotating movements 10 to 15 times.

17) Attacking one side suddenly. Stand with the feet wider than a shoulder width. Hold the left hand akimbo and stretch the right palm and lift it to its highest position. Turn the waist to the left, vibrate the hand twice and inhale twice. After that, bring down the right hand to its former position while exhaling. Change to the left hand and do the same. Repeat this routine 10 to 15 times.

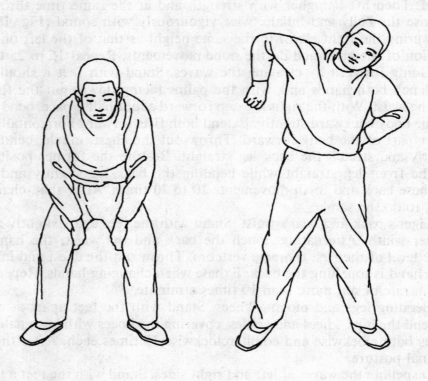

Fig. 17   Fig. 18

18) The prancing of a dragon and leaping of a tiger. Stand with the feet apart a little more than a shoulder width. Bend the knees slightly. Extend both arms to the sides of the body horizontally. Touch the right knee with the left hand, then the left knee with right hand, moving along a wheel-like line (Fig. 19). Breathe once during the rotation. Repeat in this way 10 to 15 times.

19) Fishing out a pearl from the bottom of sea. Stand with the feet a shoulder width apart. Lift the right foot 10 cm above the ground and let it make 5-cm circles, then put it down. Breathe once for each circle. Rotate 6 to 8 times. Do the same with the left foot. Repeat the routine 4 to 10 times.

20) Turning round the heaven and earth. Stand with the feet apart wider than a shoulder width. Put the left hand on the middle part of the waist, bend the knees, and rotate the right hand beginning from the middle Dantian (the pectoral region) clockwise upward to the level of the lower jaw then downward to above the knees. Breathe once for each circle. After rotating 10 to 15 circles, change to the left hand to do the same. Repeat this routine 4 to 6 times.

21) Mutual helping at the back. Stand with the feet apart wider than a shoulder

width. Throw out the chest and tense the abdomen. Breathing naturally, clasp one hand with the other on the back of the lumbar vertebra. Pull the hands to the right, then to the left as much as possible. Pull about 15 to 20 times. After that change the position of the hands and do the pull movements another 15 to 20 times. Repeat this routine 4 to 6 times.

22) Expelling waves and kicking water. Stand with the feet apart wider than a shoulder width. Push both hands backward to the left as though expelling water, at the same time turning the waist, kicking out the right leg (Fig. 20), and inhaling. Restore the former position and exhale. Repeat the movements with alternative legs 10 to 15 times.

23) Luring the dragon out of the water. Stand with the feet apart wider than a shoulder width. Swing the right arm in circular motion. Inhale when the right hand reaches the maximal height and exhale when it is falling down, swinging 10 to 15 times. Then change to the left arm in the same routine. Repeat 4 to 6 times.

24) Mutual help between firmness and gentleness. Stand with the feet apart wider than a shoulder width. With both hands akimbo, rotate the hips, turning and swivelling. Lift up the *qi* and contract the sphincter. Rotate clockwise first for 10 to 15 rounds, then counterclockwise for another 10 to 15 rounds. Breathe once for each round. Repeat routine 2 to 4 times.

25) Seizing the laurel. Stand with the feet apart at a distance less than a shoulder width. Clench the hands loosely, lifting them up and inhaling. Vibrate them twice when they reach the maximal height and inhale twice. Then bring down both hands while exhaling. Exercise 10 to 20 times.

26) Ba Wang, the conqueror, making his appearance. Stand with the feet a shoulder width apart. Droop the left hand down. Make the right hand clenched lossely and lift it up from the front to the height of the eyes and turn the palm suddenly forward, lifting the left leg and inhaling at the same time. Then restore the former position and exhale. Change to the left hand and the right leg to do the same movements. Repeat 15 to 25 times.

27) Crane hovering in the air. Stand with the feet a little wider than a shoulder width apart. Extend both arms to the sides horizontally, squat down and stand up alternatively, and flap both arms like a crane flapping its wings in flight. Bending down and standing should be the main movements, arms moving passively. Breathe once for each "flap." Repeat the movements 10 to 20 times.

28) Making a stormy sea stormier. Stand with the feet apart a little wider than a shoulder width. Retract both hands in front of the shoulders with the palms facing forward (Fig. 21). Rotate the arms from the upper side downward laterally. Breathe once for each circle. Repeat the movements 10 to 20 times.

29) Raising hands high into the sky. Stand with the feet a shoulder width apart. Clench both hands loosely, putting the left one on the back of the waist while lifting the right one up to a level slightly above the head, with the palm facing

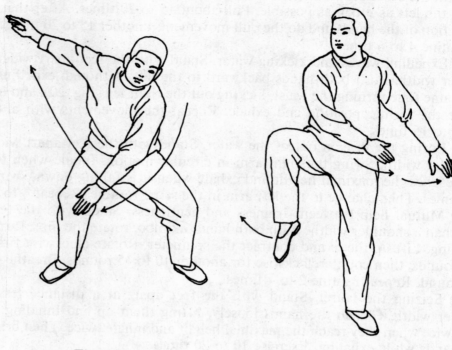

Fig. 19   Fig. 20

forward. Throw out the chest and tense the abdomen, inhaling at the same time. Then lower the right fist and put it on the back of the waist while exhaling. After that, change to the left hand to do the same movements. Repeat 10 to 20 times, at a rate of about 10 times a minute.

30) Fishing out the moon from the lake. Stand with the feet greater than a shoulder width apart. Squat down a little with left hand akimbo. Make the right hand a spoon-like form with the palm facing up and rotate it from the lateral upper side downward to the inner side, passing the knee. Thus a large circle is made as though "fishing out" the moon (Fig. 22). Then stand up and inhale. Exhale while squatting again. Repeat 10 to 15 times. After that, do these movements with the left hand. Exercise alternating hands in this way 4 to 6 times.

31) Tranquil inside while mobile outside. Stand with the feet a shoulder width apart. Press the left hand on the side of the hip, clench the right hand loosely and lift it up to the height slightly above the head with its palm facing the front. Then, vibrate the right hand backward two times and inhale twice vigourously with sound. Lower the right hand and exhale at the same time. After that, change to the left hand to do the same movements. Repeat 10 to 15 times. It is appropriate

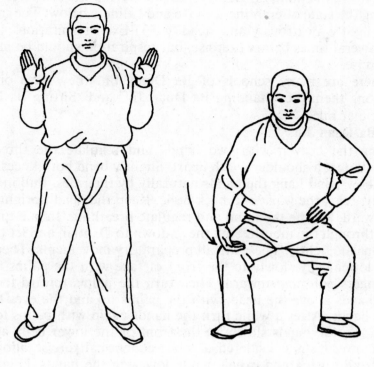

Fig. 21   Fig. 22

to do ten times a minute.

EIGHT PIECES OF BROCADE EXERCISE
(Ba Duan Jin)

Ba Duan Jin is part of the health care Qigong system practised in the home which has been popularized among Chinese people. This exercise was practised in the Sui and Tang dynasties (581-907 A.D.). It is easily performed by both old and young people. The amount of exercise can be varied and its effect is all-round. Its movements are divided into eight steps, the postures in each as graceful as a brocade, hence the name Ba Duan Jin.

The following points should be emphasized in practising this exercise: (1) Firmness and gentleness should be combined. During exercise, the muscles and nerves of the whole body have to be relaxed, movements being done by inserting force lightly and slowly. Throughout the exercise, it is required to achieve tightness within looseness, and firmness within gentleness, but never exercising with stiff force. (2) Concentrate the mind on Dantian, thus lowering the centre of gravity of the body, forming the state of emptiness above and fullness below. The movements should be done lightly, dextrously and steadily. (3) Even respiration is required. Breathe deeply several times before exercise, but respiration should be natural and even during exercise.

Although there are many schools of Ba Duan Jin, they have only minor differences. Among them the "Standing Ba Duan Jin" and "Sitting Ba Duan Jin" are the most popular ones.

1. Standing Ba Duan Jin

1) Supporting the heaven with two hands and regulate the three visceral cavities. Stand with feet a shoulder width apart. Slightly bend both knees, relax the shoulders and elbows, and hang the hands naturally by the sides. Pull in the chest, contract the belly, relax the waist and back bone. Keep the head upright, with the eyes looking forward. Soothe the mind and regulate breathing. Inhale through the nose and exhale through the mouth. Sink the *qi* down to Dantian and let the tongue touch the upper palate lightly. These are all preparatory movements. Then lift both hands from the lower belly slowly to the front of face with the palms facing the body and the fingers pointing upward. Then turn the palms toward the sky and slowly lift both hands above the head, with the palms up and the eyes looking at the backs of the hands. After a while turn the hands again with palms toward the face and bring down the hands slowly to the front of the lower belly again. One raising and one lowering is considered as one sequence. Exercise altogether six times. Inhale during raising and exhale while lowering the hands. (Figs. 23-1, 2, 3, 4)

2) Shooting first to one side, then to the other as though hunting vultures. Stand with the previous posture. Move the left foot a step horizontally to the left to form a horse-riding stance with the knees turning a little inward, the feet firmly on the ground and thighs almost level. Cross the hands in front of the chest, with the left hand outside, right hand inside and the palms facing the shoulders. Hold the fingers like the form of a sword and rotate the arms outwards. Push the left hand to the left side with its palm facing outside and the tiger's mouth (between the thumb and the index finger) up. Stretch the left arm as in the posture of shooting while turning the head to the left, with the eyes looking at the left fingers. At the same time, hold the right hand as if pulling a bowstring to the right side. Stop a while and then cross the hands again in front of the chest with the right hand outside and left hand inside. This is the left posture. The right posture is just the opposite, i.e., do the same movements with the opposite hands. One left and one right movement is considered as one sequence. Exercise six times. Finally droop both hands at the sides of the body, inhaling as you turn the head to the left and exhaling while turning it to the right (Figs. 24-1, 2, 3).

3) Regulate the function of the spleen and stomach with one arm lifting. Stand

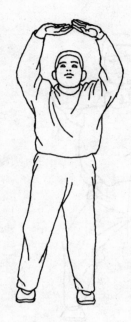

Fig. 23-1

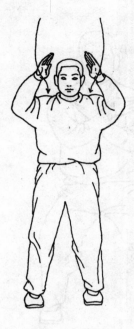

Fig. 23-2

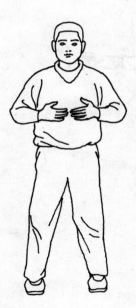

Fig. 23-3

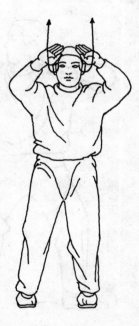

Fig. 23-4

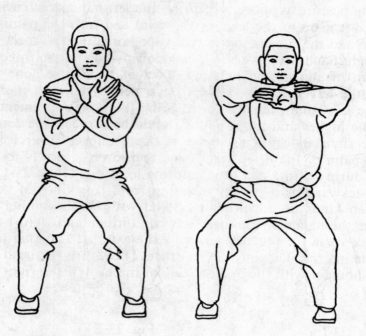

Fig. 24-1   Fig. 24-2

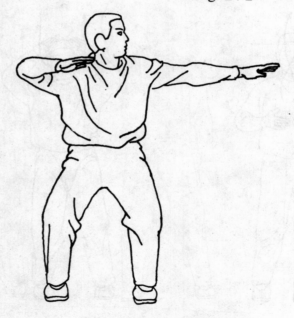

Fig. 24-3

with the beginning posture as above. Turn first the left hand slowly with its palm facing face, then lift it up to the level of the head and turn the palm upward as you turn the head and the fingers to the right side horizontally. At the same time press down the right hand with its palm facing downward and the fingers pointing to the front. Both lifting up and pressing down of hands are done with equal strength. This is the left style. The right style is performed with the right hand lifting up and the left hand pressing down, doing the same movements as in the left style. Both the higher and lower palms should be turned. The completion of one left and one right style is considered as one sequence. Exercise six times. Finally, turn the palm of the lifted right hand and lower it slowly to the side of the body. Inhale during lifting and exhale during lowering. (Figs. 25-1, 2, 3)

4) Looking backward by a person suffering from five kinds of consumptive diseases and seven kinds of impairments. Stand with the beginning posture as above. First place the hands on Dantian, left hand inside and right hand outside for males and vice-versa for females, covering the external Laogong point of the one hand with the internal Laogong of the other. Then, turn the head toward the back of the left shoulder with the eyes looking at the heel of the right foot. After

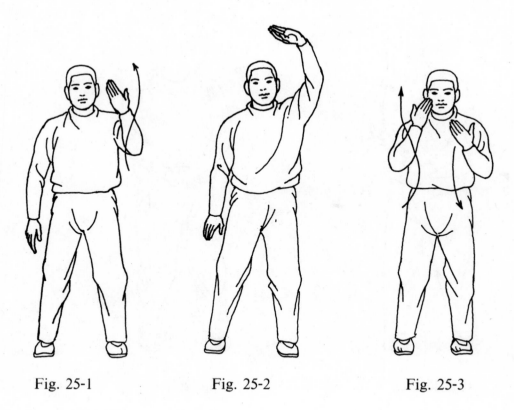

Fig. 25-1   Fig. 25-2   Fig. 25-3

stopping for a while, turn the head back with the eyes looking ahead. This is the left style. In the right style the movements are the same but with opposite direction. The completion of both one left and one right style is considered to be one sequence. Exercise altogether six times. Finally, return the hands to the sides of the body. Inhale when turning the head to the left side and exhale when turning it to the right. (Figs. 26-1, 2)

5) Expel the fire of the heart by shaking the head and wagging the tail. Stand with the posture as above. Bend the knees to form the horse riding stance. Press the hands on the thighs, with the fingers of both hands facing each other. Slant the upper part of the body forward and rotate it along an arc from the left to the right side. At the same time swing the head from left to right. This is the left style. In the right style the movements are the same but with opposite direction. The completion of both left and right styles is considered to be one sequence. Exercise altogether six times. Finally return both hands to the sides of the body. Inhale when swinging from left to right and exhale when swinging from right to left. (Figs. 27-1, 2, 3)

6) Reinforce the kidney and loins through grasping the feet with the hands.

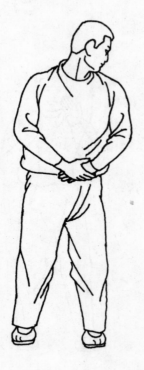

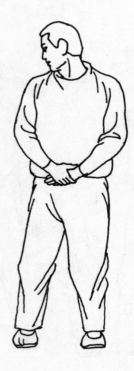

Fig. 26-1   Fig. 26-2

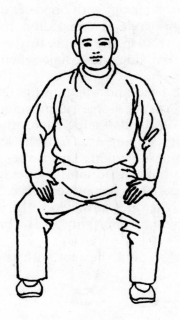

Fig. 27-1

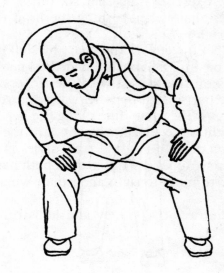

Fig. 27-2

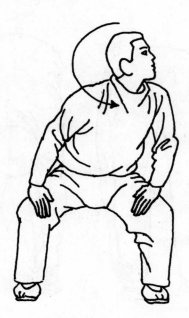

Fig. 27-3

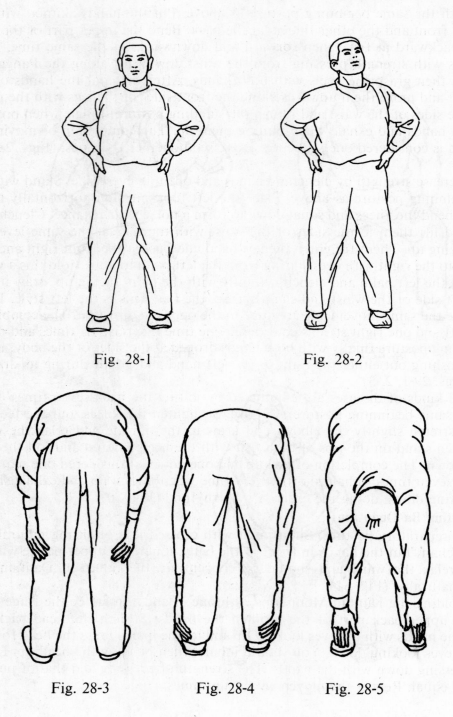

Fig. 28-1   Fig. 28-2

Fig. 28-3   Fig. 28-4   Fig. 28-5

Stand with the same beginning posture as above. Put the hands akimbo with the thumb in front and the other fingers at the back. Bend the upper part of the body slightly backward at first, then forward and downward. At the same time, move the hands with strength pressing from the waist downward along the Pangguang channels, then grasp the heels with both hands. After that put the hands on the tip of feet and move them upwards along the front sides of the legs with the palms facing the sides of the waist and return the standing posture. Inhale when pressing down the hands and exhale when pulling them up. The completion of moving up and down is considered one sequence. Exercise altogether six times. (Figs. 28-1, 2, 3, 4, 5)

7) Increase strength by clenching hands and opening eyes wide. Stand with the same beginning posture as above. Place the left foot one step horizontally to the left side, bend the knees and squat down to form a horse riding stance. Clench both hands and lift them to the sides of the waist with the fists at the same level and palms facing up. Then straighten the left hand and push it the front right and turn the head to the right with eyes staring from the left palm to afar. Hold this a while, then turn the left palm and clench it tightly with the palm facing up, draw it back to the left side of the waist and slightly relax the fist. This is the left style. In the right style the same movements are done in the opposite direction. The completion of one left and one right style is considered one time. Exercise six times and return the standing posture finally with both hands droped at the sides of the body. Inhale during pushing out either the right or the left hand and exhale during its drawing back. (Figs. 29-1, 2, 3)

8) All kinds of diseases are eliminated by jolting the back seven times. Stand with the same beginning posture as above. Straighten the knees, put the feet side by side, stretch slightly the elbows and arms to the outside and relax the whole body. Then stand on the tips of both feet with the heels relaxed and jolt the body up and down. The completion of one up and one down is considered one sequence. Exercise seven times. Inhale shortly every time when jolting up and exhale shortly when jolting down, doing the exercise with rhythm. (Fig. 30)

2. Sitting Ba Duan Jin

The preparatory posture: Sit straight with crossed legs or sitting naturally on a bed or chair. Put the hands in front of the belly, touch the upper palate with the tongue, relax the waist and shoulders, concentrate the mind on Dantian, and breathe naturally. (Fig. 31)

1) Holding the Kunlun Mountains with one's hands. Interlace the fingers and hold the upper back part of the head in the hands. Stretch the head backward against the hands with the eyes looking up and let the hands press the head forward with the eyes looking down. You should inhale when pushing the head up. Exhale when pressing down with the hands. The strength of pressing and that of pushing are to be equal. Repeat the movements many times. (Fig. 32-1)

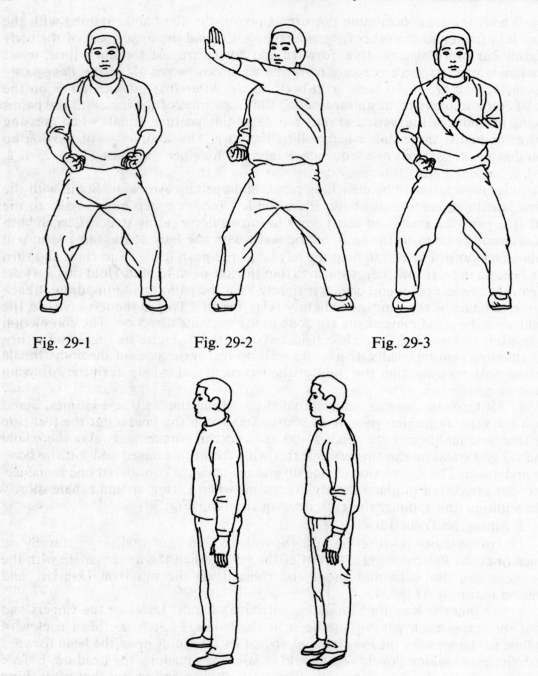

Fig. 29-1   Fig. 29-2   Fig. 29-3

Fig. 30

When the head is turning to the right, press the head with the hands to the left and let the eyes look to the right side. Then turn the head to the left, with the hands and eyes doing the same movements to the opposite sides. Inhale when looking to the left and exhale when looking to the right. Repeat many times. (Fig. 32-2)

The movements of this step are helpful mainly to strengthen the muscles of the neck and speed up the blood circulation in the top of head. However, for the hypertensive patients, this exercise should be performed in accordance with the state of their own body.

2) Shaking lightly the cervical vertebrae. Relax the muscles of the whole body. Without moving the shoulders and arms, swing the waist and the belly slightly, while the head and neck turn passively. (Figs. 33-1, 2, 3)

Turn first from left to right clockwise many times then from right to left counterclockwise many times. Infloat and contract the belly alternately along with the turning of the neck.

The exercise of this step is chiefly the moving of the waist, while the turning of the head and neck are passive movements. The peristalsis of the internal organs are reinforced, along with the movements of the muscles in the upper part of the body. It is helpful in improving blood circulation and the functions of the internal organs.

3) Supporting the sky and pressing the top of head. Lift both hands from the sides of the body to the top of head and cross the fingers. Then turn the palms up and push them up with strength until the elbows are straight. Stretch the whole body, contract the sphincter, and inhale at the same time. (Fig. 34-1)

Relax the whole body, bend both arms without turning the palms, press the top of the head lightly and exhale (Fig. 34-2). Repeat the movements of pushing and pressing in this way many times. Finally bring down hands to restore the preparatory posture.

The exercise of this step can stretch the muscles of the trunk and arms, as well as reinforce the sphincter muscle and thus is helpful in preventing and curing hemorrhoids and other diseases.

4) Grasping fast the underside of the arch of the foot. Sitting upright with both legs stretched straight, bend the upper part of the body as low as possible, lift both arms forward and horizontally, and then grasp the underside of the arch of both feet (Fig. 35-1). At the same time let the upper part of the body spring up and down for many times. (Fig. 35-2)

For beginners, move both hands towards the feet as near as possible and the forehead towards the legs as close as possible. The exercise of this step can help to stretch the muscles of the waist and the back, and reinforce the kidney and the waist.

5) Rotating a wheel with arms. Lift the arms forward and horizontally. Clench

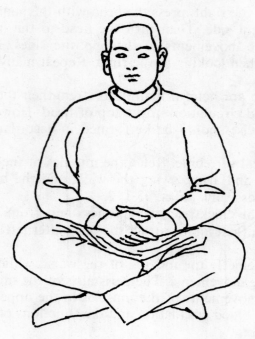

Fig. 31

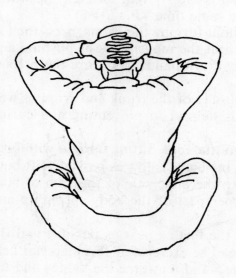

Fig. 32-1

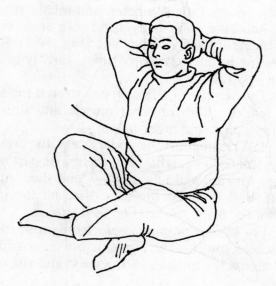

Fig. 32-2

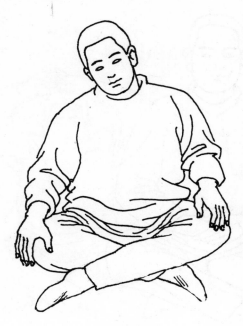

Fig. 33-1

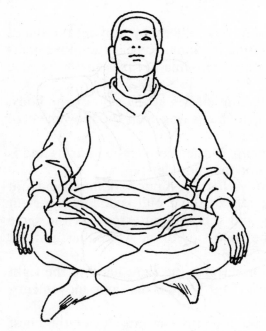

Fig. 33-2

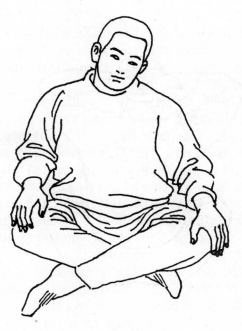

Fig. 33-3

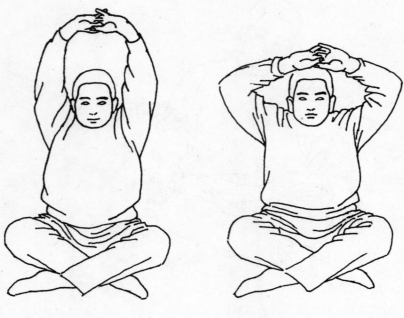

Fig. 34-1   Fig. 34-2

the hands slightly, then making circles in front of the body by moving the hands up, forward, down, backward as though rotating a winch. Repeat the movements many times (Fig. 36-1), then do the same movements many times in the reverse direction.

Do similar movements with one hand making circles at the side of the body, then the other, the head and shoulders being rocked along with the movement of the arm. (Fig. 36-2) Repeat this way many times.

This exercise mainly involves the movements of the shoulders and arms and is helpful in the prevention and cure of illness of the shoulder region.

6) Shooting first to one side and then to the other. First put both hands in front of the chest, then push the left hand to the left side and pull suddenly the right hand to the right as though drawing a bow and shooting an arrow. At the same time swing the right elbow vigorously to the right side once. After that, put the hands in front of the belly.

Lift the hands again to the front of the chest, push the right hand to the right side and pull the left hand violently to the left (Fig. 37). Do the same movements, alternating directions for many times.

The exercise of this step is helpful in strengthening the muscles of the chest and back, reinforcing the functions of the respiratory system and increasing vital

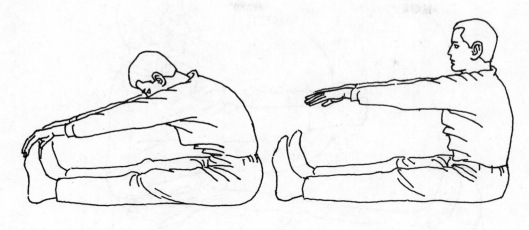

Fig. 35-1   Fig. 35-2

capacity.

7) Boxing with two hands. Clench both hands and box forward violently with the two fists alternatively for many times. (Fig. 38)

Then box the fists to the left and the right alternatively.

Cross boxing: Let the left fist box to the front-right direction and the right one to the front-left direction. Repeat in this way for many times.

8) Tapping the whole body. Clench the hands loosely and tap the whole body with them, beginning from the waist and back, then to the chest and belly, shoulders, neck, four limbs and the rest of the body.

This step is for relaxing and straightening out.

SINEW-TRANSFORMING EXERCISE
(Yi Jin Jing)

Yi Jin Jing evolved and developed from the Daoyin Fa (method of breathing and physical exercise therapy) and Tuna Fa (method of inspiration and expiration) of the ancient Yangsheng Shu (exercise for health cultivation). It is said that it was created by the eminent monk Damo of the Shaolin Temple in the Liang Dynasty (502-557 A.D.) and Chen Bo of the Song Dynasty (960-1279 A.D.) in the course of their exercises. It has been one of the methods of physical exercise beloved by Chinese people for centuries. The word "Yi" means change, "Jin" denotes the muscles and bones, and "Jing" signifies method. In other words, Yi Jin Jing refers to one of the health care methods for changing of the weak and withered muscles

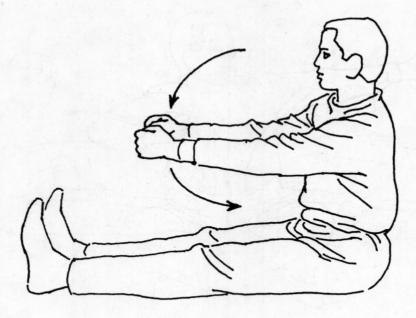

Fig. 36-1

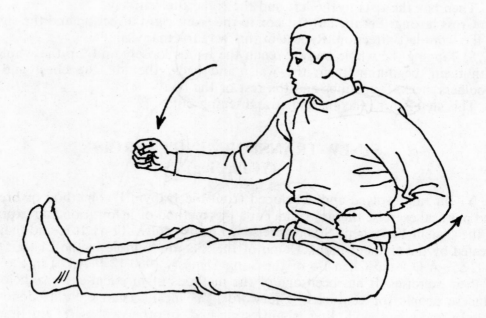

Fig. 36-2

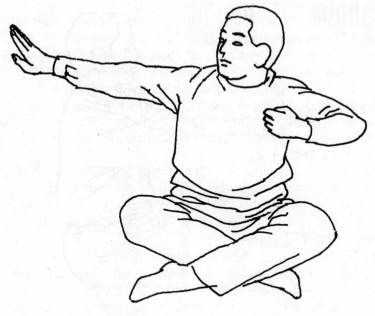

Fig. 37

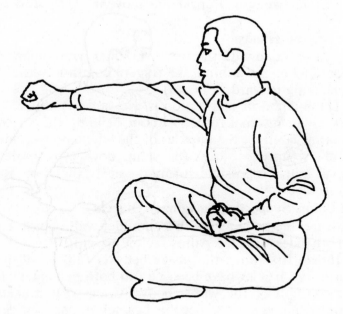

Fig. 38

and bones into strong and sturdy ones.

Yi Jin Jing is characterized by close combination of respiration with movements, putting forth strength statically (i.e., using internal force), relaxation, nature concentration of mind on Dantian, and mutual help between firmness and gentleness. The common points in the preparatory posture for perfoming the movements of each step are: looking ahead horizontally, clamping the teeth tightly, opening the mouth slightly or closing it lightly, and touching the upper palate with the tongue; no use of strength, no throwing out of the chest, no lifting of the shoulders, and no bending of the back; natural respiration, relaxing of the whole body, concentration on Dantian.

There are many schools of Yi Jin Jing. This book introduces ten steps which are simple and easy to perform. For beginners, every movement can be exercised 8 to 9 times at the start and be increased gradually to 30 times or more according to the status of the body of the exerciser along with the level of skill in practice.

1. Respiration with Clenched Hands

The preparatory posture: Stand with the feet a shoulder width apart, clench both hands with the centre of fist facing back and the tip of thumbs touching the thighs. (Fig. 39)

Exercise method: breathe softly with the abdominal respiration method. Infloat the belly during inhalation. Clench the hands tightly during exhalation and don't open the fists at the next inhalation. During the next exhalation, clench the hands more tightly with increasing strength. Repeat the movements several times this way.

2. Respiration with Pressed Hands

The preparatory posture: Stand with the feet a shoulder width apart. Drop the hands with the palms parallel to the ground, the fingers pointing to the sides, and the tips of the fingers bending upward. (Fig. 40)

Exercise method: The method of respiration is the same as above except the palms are pressing down with internal force (without bending the knees) during exhalation. At the same time contract the muscles of the whole body gradually and keep the tensive state of the muscles. Press the palms down with more strength and bend the fingers up as much as possible during the next exhalation. Repeat the movement many times in this way.

3. Respiration with Palms Supporting Imaginary Objects

The preparatory posture: Separate feet with a shoulder width apart and lift the hands horizontally to both sides with the palms facing up. (Fig. 41)

Exercise method: Inhale first until the lower belly is fully swollen. During exhalation imagine that heavy articles have been put on both palms which need to be supported with the strength of the whole body. Along with exhalation, the imagined supported objects should seem to become heavier and heavier demanding ever stronger internal force. It should be noted that the position of both hands is not to be changed. Repeat the movements many times in this way.

4. Respiration with the Bracing Palms

The preparatory posture: Separate the feet with a shoulder width apart, lift both hands horizontally at both sides and bend the wrist upward with the palms facing out. The fingers should be bent with strength toward the head to form a posture as though were bracing something against the air by both palms. (Fig. 42)

Exercise method: The method of respiration is the same as above. During exhalation, brace both palms to the sides with internal strength as though pushing objects away. Cause the muscles of the whole body to be in a tensive state gradually along with the pushing movements. The "strength" of the pushing should become stronger as the imagined objects are pushed farther and farther. Repeat several times in this way. (Fig. 42)

5. Respiration with Hands Joining and Separating

The preparatory posture: Separate the feet with a shoulder width apart. Join the palms of the hands in front of the chest with the thumbs touching the chest. (Fig. 43-1)

Exercise method: During inhalation, keep both elbows at the same level,

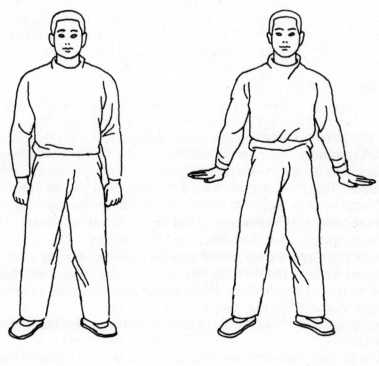

Fig. 39   Fig. 40

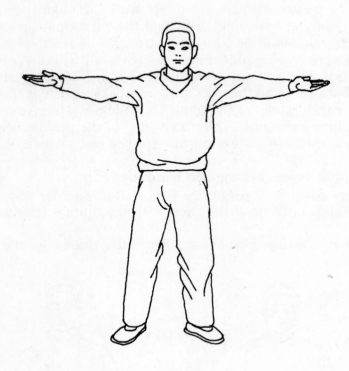

Fig. 41

separate the palms slowly to both sides of the chest with the thumbs moving along the chest. Gradually tense up the muscles of the whole body along with the moving of the hands (Fig. 43-2). During exhalation let both palms return slowly to the joining state. The movements should be done along with the respiration and the breath should be slow, relaxed, quiet, soft and even. Repeat many times in this way.

6. Respiration with a Bracing Hand and a Dropping Hand

The preparatory posture: Place the left leg to the left to form the left bow stance with the right leg stretched straight, straighten the body naturally, lift up the left hand with its palm facing up. At the same time drop the right hand to the right side of the body with its palm stretched straight and facing the thigh and the fingers pointing down. (Fig. 44-1)

Exercise method: No change of the position of the body in the whole process of respiration.

During respiration, prop up the left hand with internal strength and drop the right hand as though wanting to draw the distance between the hands longer.

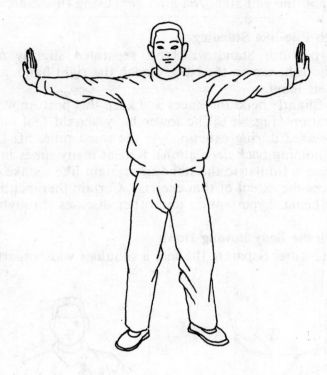

Fig. 42

Contract the muscles of the whole body along with the movements. Repeat several times in this way, relaxing the body naturally.

Change to the right bow stance and do the same movements of propping up and droping down in the opposite direction. (Fig. 44-2).

7. Respiration with the Body Moving Up and Down

The preparatory posture: Stand naturally with the feet apart at a shoulder width.

Exercise method: Lift up both arms forward horizontally from the lower side. Bend both arms naturally with the palms facing up (Fig. 45-1). Then, turn the palms downward and at the same time squat down slowly with the upper part of the body straight (Fig. 45-2). The extent of squatting can be increased day by day until the thighs can come parallel to the ground. Turn the palms again upward, lifting up the body slowly (Fig. 45-3), and return the original position. Then turn the palms once more and get ready to squat. (Fig. 45-4)

In this exercise, inhale when lifting the hands and exhale when squatting and turning the hands. Repeat many times in this way. The waist can be strengthened, the kidney fastened, and the gait stablized after practising this exercise for a long period.

8. Respiration with Pile-like Standing

The preparatory posture: Stand with feet separated slightly more than a shoulder width. Put both hands on the back, clench the right hand, and grasp the right wrist with the left hand.

Exercise method: Slightly bend the knees and keep this posture while performing abdominal respiration (Fig. 46). The lower belly should feel bloated during inhalation and compressed during exhaling. At the same time, lift the anus (i.e. exercise it as though holding back defecation). Repeat many times in this way.

This step of exercise is similar to the standing straight like a stake exercise, and in some ways reinforces the extent of that exercise. Certain therapeutic effects can be gained for neurasthenia, hypertention and other diseases through performing it.

9. Respiration with the Body Bowing Down

The preparatory posture: Separate the feet a shoulder width apart. (Fig. 47-1)

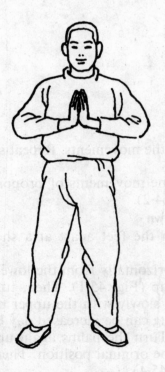

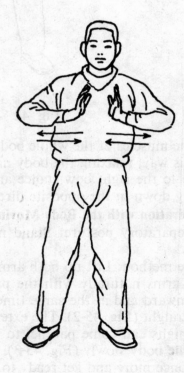

Fig. 43-1   Fig. 43-2

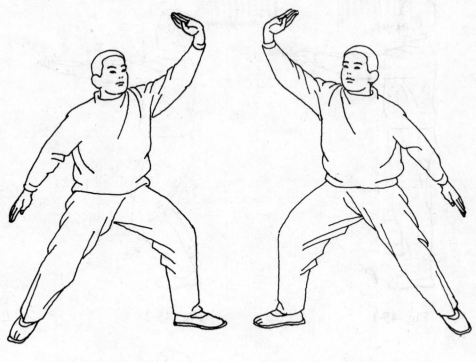

Fig. 44-1   Fig. 44-2

Exercise method: Bend the upper part of the body forward slowly to an angle of 90 degrees. At the same time, drop both hands as you loosen and lightly move about the shoulders. Let the palms face the body and fingers point at the ground (Fig. 47-2). The hands should be relaxed without putting forth strength. Exhale when bending the body and inhale when straightening. Repeat several times in this way.

This step of the exercise is helpful to eliminate excess belly fat and relieve backaches and pain in the waist.

10. Respiration with Twisting of the Body and Looking About

Exercise method: 1) Place the left foot a large step to the left side to form a left bow stance. After twisting the body leftwise, put the left hand on the waist with the palm facing outward. Put the right hand in front of the forehead at a distance of one fist, with its palm facing outward and eyes looking at the right heel. Do not raise the heel from the ground (Fig. 48-1). When the left bow stance is exercised, the waist is in a tensive state due to the twisting of the body to the left. Imagine that the centre of gravity of the body is transferred to the right heel when exhaling. The extent of twisting of the waist should be inereased gradually.

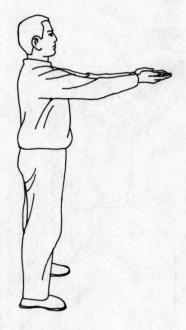

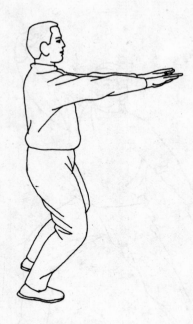

Fig. 45-1   Fig. 45-2

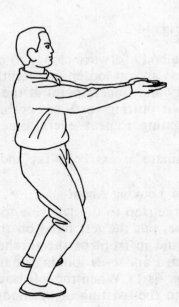

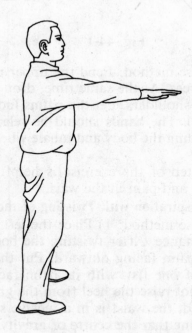

Fig. 45-3   Fig. 45-4

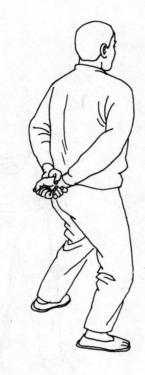

Fig. 46

It is best to practise abdominal respiration for this step.

2) The movements in the right bow stance are the same as those above except the direction is opposite. (Fig. 48-2)

It is helpful for the prevention of back pain after frequent exercise.

THE BUDDHA'S GUARDIANS' EXERCISE
(Jin Gang Gong)

According to legend, Jin Gang Gong was created by a general of the Qing Dynasty (1644-1911 A.D.). This general was proficient in both Qigong and medical skills. He later shaved his head and became a monk. This school of exercise was established by successors through selection. It consists of three steps. As with other exercises, it stresses the regulation of the heart, the body and the breath. The exercise should be done with relaxed body and soft breath, and without distracting thoughts.

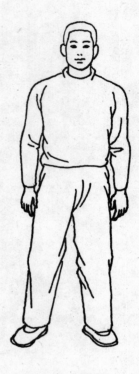

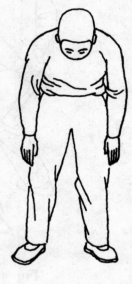

Fig. 47-1   Fig. 47-2

1. Exercise Method

1) The first step

a. The preparatory posture: Put both hands on the lower belly one and a half *cun* below the navel with the right hand covering the left one, both thumbs opposing each other and the palms facing up. Breathe three times. (Fig. 49-1)

b. Hold the hands parallel to the ground with the palms facing up and lift them to the chest. Inhale when lifting of the hands. (Fig. 49-2)

c. Turn the palms downward and drop them down slowly to the sides of the body until both arms are straight. Exhale. (Fig. 49-3)

d. Move both hands away from the body and lift them up to the level of the eyebrows, with the palms facing the body. Inhale when lifting the hands. Then turn the hands inwards so that the palms now face outward. Exhale when turning the hands. (Fig. 49-4)

e. Stretch both arms straight to the sides at the level of the shoulders, with the palms still facing outward. Inhale while stretching the arms and lift the anus once.

Then turn the elbows to the sides with the palms facing out. Exhale while turning the palms. (Fig. 49-5)

   f. Turn the body to the left with the left foot forward front and the right one behind. The distance between the feet should be a shoulder width. Clench both hands while turning the body, with the thumbs put inside the centre of the fist and the other four fingers covering it on the outside. Put the fists on the place between the back and the waist with the back of the hands facing the body. Breathe once. Then lift both fists slowly to the ribs of both sides and breathe once more. After that return the preparatory posture and repeat the movements of parts (1) to (5) and breathe. Then do the same movements of part (6) in the opposite direction. (Fig. 49-6)

   g. Turn the body to the right with the right foot at front and the left one at back. The distance between the feet should be a shoulder width. Clench the hands while turning the body and put them on the place between the back and the waist with the back of the fists facing the body. Breathe once, then lift the fists to the ribs of both sides and breathe once again. After that, return to the preparatory posture. Repeat the movements alternately three times. Then rub the chest (rub

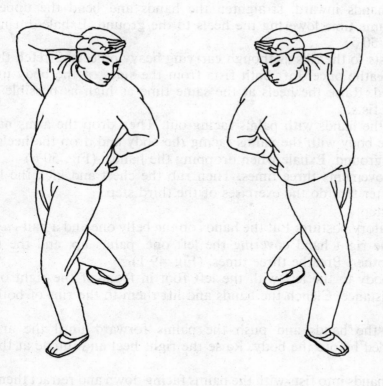

Fig. 48-1   Fig. 48-2

the front part of the chest with one palm first and then with the other) and kick the legs (lift one foot and kick it out slowly, and then do the same movement with another foot) for three minutes. After that do the exercises of the second step.

2) The second step

a. The preparatory posture: Do the movements of parts (1) to (4) of the first step, then bend both arms and the upper part of the body forward slowly. The distance between the arms should be a shoulder width, and the palms facing inside. Exhale during bending. (Fig. 50-1)

b. Clench both hands as though they were carrying very heavy objects and lift them along the legs to the ribs, then breathe once. Raise both fists upward from the sides of the body until the arms are straight. Raise the heels as high as possible. Inhale when lifting the fists. (Fig. 50-2)

c. Bring the fists along the head and over the ears to the ribs. At the same time squat slowly and keep the heels raised. Exhale when bringing down the fists. (Fig. 50-3)

d. Straighten the hands and push the palms forward until the arms are completely extended before the body. Inhale when pushing. (Fig. 50-4)

e. Turn the hands inward, straighten the hands and bend the upper body forward, at the same time lowering the heels to the ground. Exhale during these movements. (Fig. 50-5)

f. Lift both fists to the ribs as though carrying heavy objects. Stretch the body straight. Then breathe once. Lift both fists from the sides of the body until the arms are stretched. Raise the heels at the same time as high as possible. Inhale during lifting the fists.

g. Straighten the hands with palms facing out. Then drop the arms naturally to the sides of the body with the palms facing the body and drop the heels at the same time to the ground. Exhale when dropping the hands. (Fig. 50-6)

Repeat the movements three times. Then rub the chest and kick the legs for three minutes. After that do the exercises of the third step.

3) The third step

a. The preparatory posture: Put the hands on the belly one and a half *cun* below the navel with the right hand covering the left one, palms up, and the thumbs pointing at each other. Breathe three times. (Fig. 49-1)

b. Turn the body to the left with the left foot in front of the right one at a shoulder width distance. Clench the hands and lift them to the ribs of both sides. (Fig. 51-1)

c. Straighten the hands and push the palms forward until the arms are completely extended before the body. Raise the right heel and inhale at the same time. (Fig. 51-2)

d. Clench the hands into fists with the palms facing down and retract them to the ribs slowly. Drop the right heel when retracting. At the same time exhale. (Fig. 51-3)

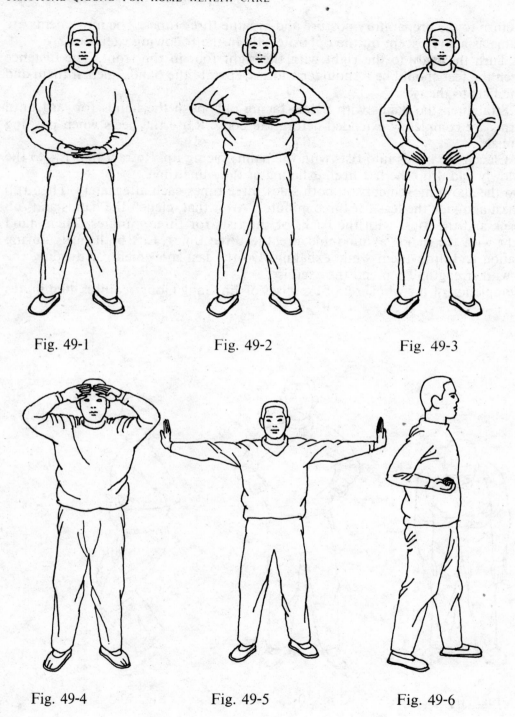

Fig. 49-1   Fig. 49-2   Fig. 49-3

Fig. 49-4   Fig. 49-5   Fig. 49-6

Return to the preparatory posture and breathe three times. The movements are the same as above except on the opposite side in the following exercises.

e. Turn the body to the right with the right foot in the front. The distance between the feet should be a shoulder width. Separate the hands, clench them and lift the fists to the ribs.

f. Straighten the hands with palms facing out, push the hands forward until the arms are completely extended before the body. Raise the heels when pushing and inhale.

g. Clench the hands into fists with the palms facing up. Retract the fists to the ribs slowly and drop the left heel, exhaling at the same time.

Do the above movements on both sides three times each alternately. Then rub the chest and kick the legs for three minutes. After that, clench the hands and rub the back and the waist with the backs of the fists for three minutes. Then stand straight with the hands akimbo and breathe three times. Lift both heels during inhalation and drop them while exhaling. Do the last movement of droping the heels with strength. Then end the exercise.

Completion of the whole set of exercises of Jin Gang Gong requires 40 minutes

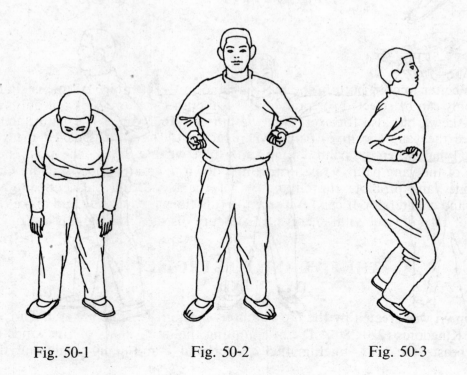

Fig. 50-1   Fig. 50-2   Fig. 50-3

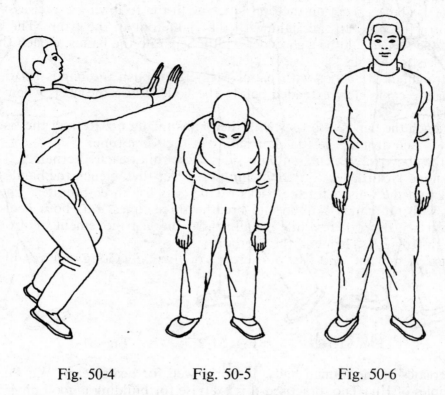

Fig. 50-4   Fig. 50-5   Fig. 50-6

or so. It is better to do it both in the morning and in the evening. If time is short, one step only can be selected for practice. This method of exercise is not only for exercising the *qi*, but also for exercising the muscles and bones. The palm facing up is called the yang (positive) palm, when facing the ground is called the yin (negative). Inhale when the palm is yang and exhale when it is yin. The *qi* is rising up in case of the yang palm, while it is falling down in case of the yin palm. One yin and one yang promote the circulation of the blood and clear up Jingluo (channels and collaterals). It can reinforce the functions of the body and make the body full of *zhen qi* (true vital energy). It can cure diseases, strengthen health.

THE FIVE ANIMALS FROLIC
(Wu Qin Xi)

Wu Qin Xi was created by the most famous master of medicine, Hua Tuo, of the Three Kingdoms (220-280 A.D.) by imitating the movements of five kinds of bird and beast—the bear, tiger, monkey, deer and crane—and combining the

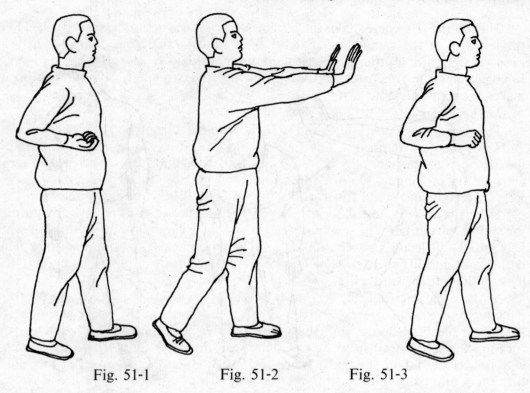

Fig. 51-1   Fig. 51-2   Fig. 51-3

characteristics of the human body. It works well for health care. Wu Pu, one of the disciples of Hua Tuo, practised this exercise for building a good physique and he could hear and see well, had firm teeth and looked like a middle-aged man even when he was more than ninety.

The Five Animals Frolic requires the exerciser to relax the whole body, to have firmness within gentleness and tightness within looseness, to concentrate the mind on Dantian, to make the upper part of the body empty while the lower part full, to breathe naturally and to perform it resembling the natural and vivid movements of the five animals both in external form and in spirit. There are many schools of Wu Qin Xi. We are going to introduce a set of movements which is rather simple and is suitable for the elderly and the weak or beginners.

1. The Bear

The preparatory posture: Stand with the feet a shoulder width apart. Drop the arms naturally. Breathe deeply 3 to 5 times (Fig. 52-1). Then do the following movements:

1) Bend the right knee, shake the right shoulder forward and downward, and lower the right arm at the same time. Extend the left shoulder backward slightly and raise the left arm a little. (Fig. 52-2)

2) Bend the left knee, shake the left shoulder forward and downward, and lower the left arm at the same time. Extend the right shoulder backward slightly and raise the right arm a little. Repeat this shaking in this way several times. (Fig. 52-3) It invigorates the functions of the spleen and the stomach, helps digestion and makes the joints flexible.

2. The Tiger

The preparatory posture: Stand with heels close, drop the shoulders naturally and erect the neck naturally. The face should have a natural expression with eyes looking forward horizontally. Close the mouth and touch the upper palate lightly with the tip of tongue. Do not throw out the chest or arch the back. (Fig. 53-1) Relax the body and stand for a while, then do the following movements.

1) Left style a. Bend the legs slowly into a posture of half squatting and move the weight of the body to the right leg. Left foot close to the right ankle with its heel raised a little and its sole touching the ground lightly. At the same time clench both hands and lift them to the sides of the waist with the palms facing up. Eyes look at the left forward. (Fig. 53-2)

b. Move the left foot one step to the left front and then move the right foot a half step to the same direction of the left foot. Let both heels face each other with a distance of about 33 cm. Let the weight of the body fall on the right leg, thus forming the left empty step. At the same time lift both fists up along the chest with fist centres facing the body. When the fists come up to the front of the mouth, turn them into palms and push them forward at the level of the chest and the eyes look at the tip of left index finger. (Fig. 53-3)

2) Right style a. Place the left foot a half step forward and then move the right foot to the left ankle joint. Keep both legs close to each other. Lift up the right heel slightly with the right sole touching the ground lightly. Bend both knees and squat a little to put the weight of the body on the left leg. At the same time clench the hands and retract them to the sides of the waist with the palms facing up and the eyes looking the right front. (Fig. 54-1)

b. Do the same movements as part (b) of the left style in the opposite direction. (Fig. 54-2)

Repeat the "tiger pouncing" movements to the right and left alternately for an unfixed number of times. It is beneficial to enhance the physical strength.

3. The Monkey

The preparatory posture is the same as that for the tiger

1) Bend both legs down slowly, move the left foot forward nimbly, lift the left hand up at the same time along the chest to the level of the mouth and then push it forward as though it were fetching an object. When the left arm is almost stretched, clench the hand and then bend the wrist downward naturally. (Fig. 55-1)

2) Place the right foot forward nimbly and then move the left foot to that direction a little. Raise the left heel, with the sole touching the ground lightly. At

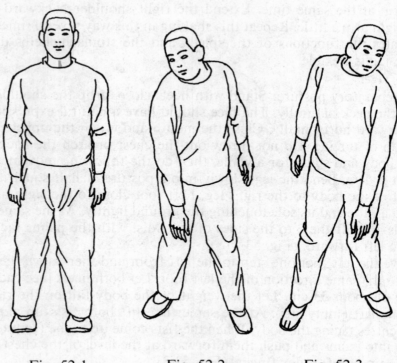

Fig. 52-1   Fig. 52-2   Fig. 52-3

the same time, lift the right hand along the chest to the level of the mouth. Then push it forward as though fetching an object. When the right arm is almost stretched, clench the hand and then bend the right wrist downward naturally. Move the left hand to the left ribs at the same time. (Fig. 55-2)

3) Draw the left foot back a little, let it touch the ground firmly and put the body weight on the left leg. Then, retreat the right foot a little with its tip touching the ground lightly. At the same time lift the left hand along the chest to the level of the mouth. Then push it forward as though fetching something. When the left arm is almost stretched, clench the hand and then bend the wrist downward naturally. Move the right hand at the same time to the ribs. (Fig. 55-3)

4) to 6) Do the same movements as those of 1) to 3) in the opposite direction (Figs. 55-4, 5). To practise this exercise is beneficial for relaxing the muscles and tendons, promoting blood circulation and enhancing the agility of the exerciser.

4. The Deer

The preparatory posture is the same as that for the tiger.

1) Bend the right leg, sit the upper part of the body backward. Move the left leg forward with its knee bent slightly and the left foot touching the ground lightly

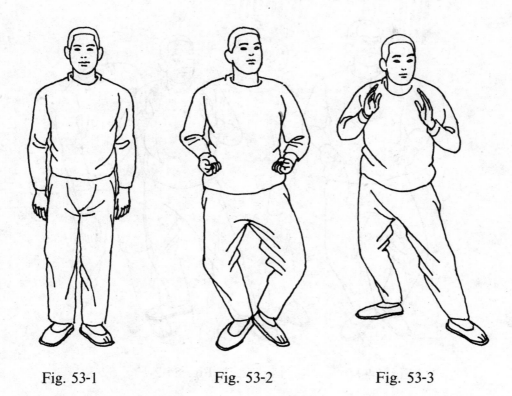

Fig. 53-1   Fig. 53-2   Fig. 53-3

to form the left empty step.

2) Stretch the left hand forward, bend the left elbow slightly and put the right hand at the inner side of the left elbow with both palms facing each other.

3) Rotate both arms counterclockwise simultaneously in front of the body. The circles made by the left hand are larger than those made by the right hand. The circular movements of the arms are brought along by the rotation of the waist and the hip, not the shoulders. The arms make larger circles while the coccyx makes smaller ones. (Fig. 56)

(4) After rotating in this way a number of times, place the right leg forward and sit the upper part of the body on the left leg. Stretch the right hand forward and put the left hand at the inner side of the right elbow. Rotate both arms clockwise simultaneously a number of times. Repeat the movements in alternating directions. This exercise is beneficial for relaxing and extending the muscles, tendons and bones.

5. The Crane

The preparatory posture: Stand with both feet close. Drop the arms naturally. LooK forward horizontally. Stand a while calmly, then do the following movements.

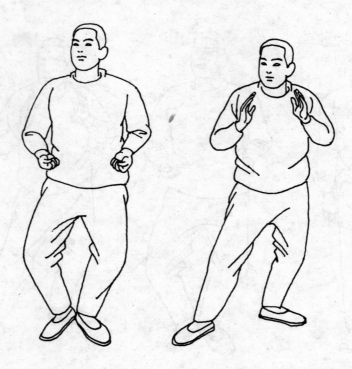

Fig. 54-1   Fig. 54-2

1) Place the left foot one step forward, then move the right foot a half step forward with the tips of the toes touching the ground lightly. At the same time lift both arms from the front of the body to the sides and inhale deeply. (Fig. 57-1)

2) Put the right foot at the side of the left one, squat down, drop both arms naturally at the sides of the body and join the forearms below the knees. Exhale deeply at the same time. (Fig. 57-2)

3) and 4) Do the same movements as in parts (1) and (2) except in the opposite direction (Fig. 57-3). This exercise is helpful for strengthening the respiratory function of the lungs, stimulating the *qi* and blood, and expelling blockage in channels and collaterals.

HARMONIZATION EXERCISE
(Tiao He Gong)

Tiao He Gong is an auxiliary exercise practised after ending of Qigong. It can be used for prevention of side-effects during performing Qigong. It was created

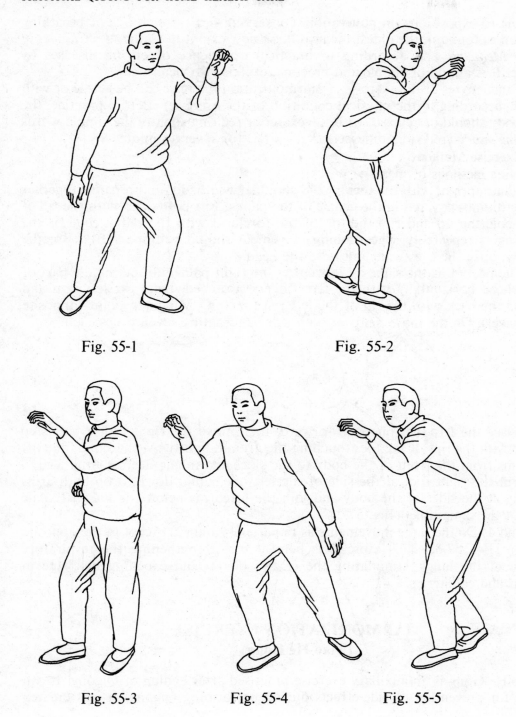

Fig. 55-1   Fig. 55-2

Fig. 55-3   Fig. 55-4   Fig. 55-5

according to expositions on cultivation, conserving health, methods of breathing and so on as found in the oldest medical book now extant in China, the *Classics of Internal Medicine*, and according to practical experience of curing diseases by massage. It is a kind of simple and practical exercise for health care.

The maneuvres of the exercise of Harmonization Exercise can be gentle or with strength, according to the physical condition of the exerciser. Before practice, the whole body should be relaxed, with the exerciser reciting silently the simple words *song—jing—song* (relaxing, quiescence, relaxing) for several minutes.

1. Exercise Method

1) Nine methods of massage

a. Stand upright with the feet spread shoulder width. Join both palms together with the thumbs covered in the centre of the palms. Lift both arms with the tip of fingers pointing up and rub the top of the forehead with the radial edge of the index fingers repeatedly. The rubbing movement should be done softly. Breathe naturally, open the eyes wide and raise the head.

b. The posture is the same as above. Let the right palm rub the middle part of the forehead horizontally with the five fingers stretched. Bend the left arm and put it on the back with the tip of the left fist touching Mingmen point (opposite to the navel). Do the movements at both sides alternating seven times each.

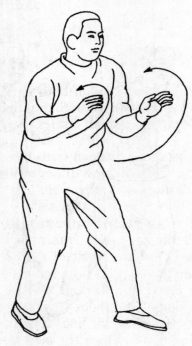

Fig. 56

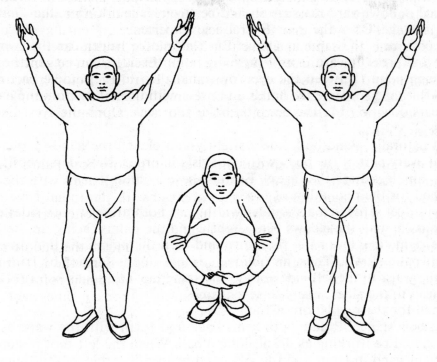

Fig. 57-1   Fig. 57-2   Fig. 57-3

c. The posture is the same as above. Clench both hands tightly. Let the tip of the second knuckle of the index fingers press on Sizhukong point (the hollow area at the lateral end of eyebrows) and make small circles there. Open the eyes. Do the movements seven times.

d. The posture is the same as above. Clench both hands as tightly as possible. Protrude the knuckle of the thumbs and press them on the orbits. Open the eyes and rub the orbits in circular motion. The directions for the left hand are upper, left, down, right, upper again. Make seven circles each.

e. The posture is the same as above. With the palms facing downward, press both thumbs with strength on Taiyang point (the hollow area behind the point where the tip of eyebrow meets the lateral angle of the eye) of both sides and rub them back and downward. Open the eyes. Do the movements seven times.

f. The posture is the same as above. Massage or rub lightly Renzhong point below the nose with the radial side of the index finger of one hand while rubbing Fengfu point (1.5 cm above the posterior hair line) with the other index finger. Do the same movements, alternating hands. Open the eyes. Exercise seven times.

g. The posture is the same as above. Place the earlobes between the index and the middle fingers of both hands. Massage with the palms up and down. The strength used in downward massage should be stronger and longer than that used in upward massage. Open the eyes. Exercise seven times.

h. The posture is the same as above. Put the middle fingers on the two sides of the nose and press upward from Yingxiang point (beside the wings of the nose) to the Yintang point (between the eyebrows) and then to the middle part of the forehead. After that, separate the hands and press with the palms from the hairline above the ears downward to the occipital bone and neck. Open the eyes. Exercise seven times.

i. Stand naturally. Bend both knees slightly and clench the hands at the same time. Pound every part of the body with both fists in order: shoulders, chest, belly, waist, back, hip, legs and other areas. Exercise seven times.

2) Method for the regulation of blood
Stand with feet separated a shoulder width. Lift both arms at both sides of the body horizontally with the elbows bent slightly and the palms facing up. Bend the waist to the right side, lower the right arm and turn the palms. At the same time raise the left palm slowly. Thus, an oblique straight line is formed by both arms. Then bow the waist to the left side and do the same movements as before. Do not swing the head to the sides. Exercise seven times.

3) Method for the regulation of food
Stand in bow stance. Rotate both arms back and forth with the waist as axis. The hands should be working as if kneading a ball. When the left foot is stepping, rotate the right hand in front and the left hand behind. Exercise seven times.

4) Method for the regulation of *qi*
Stand with feet a shoulder width apart. Stretch both arms to the sides. Bow the waist, bend the knees and squat down. At the same time, draw the hands to the front of the chest slowly to form a posture as though holding a ball. Then, stand up like a wild goose going to fly, with the arms stretching upward and separate both hands in front at the top of the head (one hand height) making again the posture of holding a ball. One squatting and one standing up is considered a sequence. Exercise altogether seven times.

TAIJI QIGONG

The Taiji Qigong follows the principle of harmonization between yin and yang, *dong* (mobility) and *jing* (quiescence) and is practised with the waist as the axis. The tissues and organs of the body can be mobilized by doing the exercise. The movements of the Taiji Qigong are simple and easy to learn. It has good effects on health strengthening. It can be exercised by anyone who can stand up.

1. The Beginning Posture and the Regulation of Breath
The preparatory posture: Stand naturally with the feet a shoulder width apart.

Keep the upper part of the body erect with the eyes looking forward horizontally. Pull in the chest, straighten the back and drop both hands naturally. (Fig. 58-1)

1) Exercise method

a. Raise the arms forward slowly until both hands are slightly above the shoulders with the palms facing down. Inhale at the same time. (Fig. 58-2)

b. Keep the upper part of the body erect. Bend both knees to an angle of about 150°. Do not protrude the kneecaps beyond the feet. Press the hands down lightly to the level of the navel with the palms facing the ground. Exhale at the same time. (Fig. 58-3)

2) Essentials

Lower the shoulders and drop down both elbows. Bend the fingers slightly and naturally. Let the weight of the body fall between the legs. Do not protrude buttocks. The movements of the arms and the body should be harmonized. Inhale when raising the hands, and exhale when they fall. One exhalation and one inhalation is considered one sequence. Exercise five times. End by putting the hands at both sides of the body.

2. Broadening the Heart and Mind

1) Exercise method

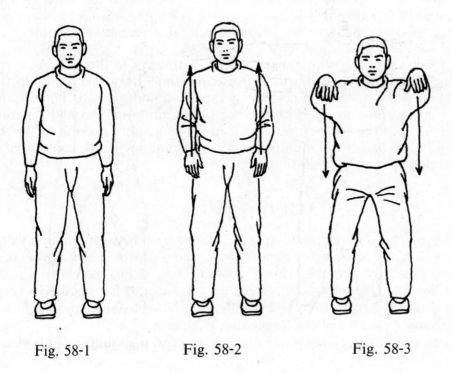

Fig. 58-1   Fig. 58-2   Fig. 58-3

a. Raise both hands, which are pressing downward, to the front of the chest while straightening the knees gradually with the palms facing each other. Pull the hands to both sides horizontally for expanding the chest. Inhale at the same time. (Fig. 59-1)

b. Remove both hands from the sides of the body horizontally to the front of the chest, with the palms facing down. Then press the hands downward while bending the knees. Exhale at the same time. (Fig. 59-2)

2) Essentials

Stand up gradually when straightening the arms and lifting them to the front of the chest and begin to squat when pressing down both hands. The movements of lifting and standing up, pressing and squatting down, inhalation and exhalation, should be done continuously.

One inhalaiton and one exhalation is considered one sequence. Exercise ten times.

3. Waving the Rainbow

1) Exercise method

a. Lift the pressing hands up to the front of the chest and at the same time stretch the knees gradually. Continue to lift both hands to the top of the head and stretch the arms straight with the palms facing the front. Inhale at the same time.

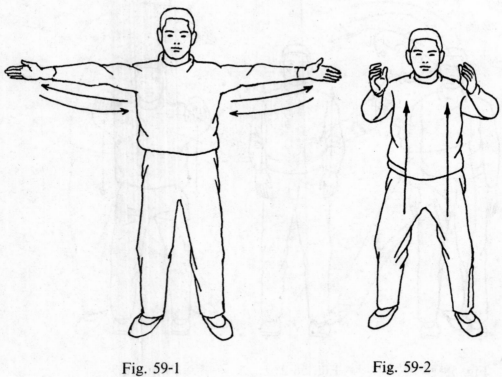

Fig. 59-1   Fig. 59-2

b. Shift the weight of the body to the right foot and bend the right leg slightly with the sole of the right foot pressing the ground. Straighten the left leg with the toes of the left foot touching the ground. Stretch the right arm from the top of the head to the left side with the right palm facing up. Bend the left elbow to form a half circle with the left palm facing down. These are the movements of the right side. Exhale at the same time. (Fig. 60-1)

c. Shift the weight of the body to the left foot, put the sole of the left foot on the ground and bend the left leg slightly. Stretch the right leg with the toes of the right foot touching the ground. Stretch the left arm from the top of head to the right side with the left palm facing up. Bend the right elbow gradually to form a half circle with the right palm facing down. These are the movements of the left side. Inhale at the same time. (Fig. 60-2)

2) Essentials

The waving movements of the hands should be soft and coordinated with the respiratory.

One inhalation and one exhalation is considered one sequence. Exercise ten

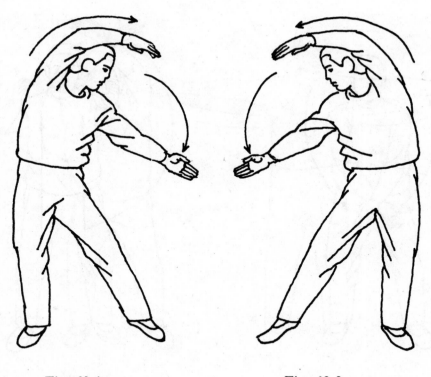

Fig. 60-1   Fig. 60-2

times.

4. Wielding the Arms for Scattering the Cloud

1) Exercise method

a. Bend both legs to form a horse riding stance and put the weight of the body between the legs. Drop the left hand from the upper left and the right one from the upper right, and cross them in front of the lower belly with the right wrist above the left one and the palms facing the body. (Fig. 61-1)

b. Straighten the legs while turning the palms up. Keep the hands crossed and lift them up to the top of head with the palms facing backward. Inhale when lifting up the hands. (Fig. 61-2)

c. Turn the palms to face outward, stretch both arms, and at the same time drop down the hands with their palms facing downward. Cross the hands gradually in front of the lower belly. Bend the elbows slightly. Exhale at the same time.

2) Essentials

Wield arms to make two large circles with the shoulder joints as the axis. When the hands are above the top of the head, the exerciser can raise the head and throw out the chest in order to help breathing. Stretch the knees while inhalation and

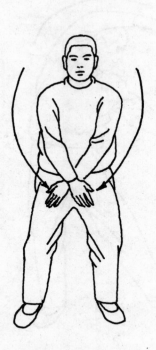

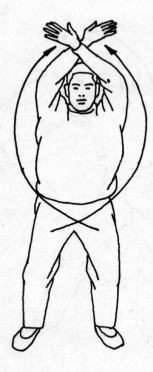

Fig. 61-1   Fig. 61-2

bend them while exhalation.

Exercise ten times.

5. Back Rolling of the Upper Arm in a Fixed Stance

1) Exercise method

a. Stand in the horse riding stance. Turn the palms of the hands, crossed in front of the lower belly, to face up. Separate the hands with the left one stretching up left and the right one lifting from the front of the belly back up along an arched line until at the horizontal position. Turn the waist to the right, let the eyes look at the right hand and inhale at the same time. Then, bend the right elbow and push the right hand forward by passing the ear with the palm facing the front. Exhale at the same time. Then, retract left hand to the front of the chest horizontally and let it come just across the hypothenar of the right hand. (Fig. 62-1)

b. Continue to lift the left hand back up along an arched line until it parallels the ground, turn the waist to the left with the eyes looking at the left hand, inhaling at the same time. Then lift the left arm, bend its elbow and push the left hand forward by passing the left ear with the palm facing the front. Exhale at the same time. Then retract right hand to the front of the chest and let it come just across the hypothenar of the left hand. (Fig. 62-2)

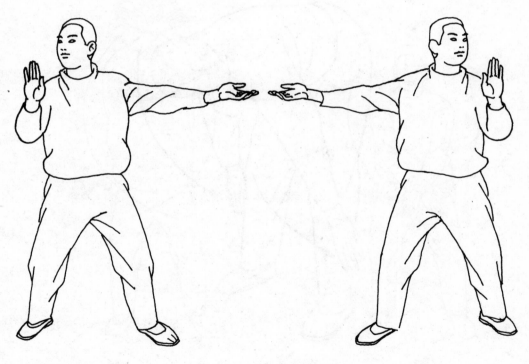

Fig. 62-1   Fig. 62-2

2) Essentials

Inhale when retracting the hand and exhale when pushing the hand.

Exercise ten times.

6. Rowing the Boat in the Lake Centre

1) Exercise method

a. When the left hand comes across the right hand in front of the chest, turn both palms up and make arched lines in front of the belly from the down to the up. Lift both arms up and stretch them, the palms facing front. Straighten the legs and inhale at the same time.

b. Make arched lines back down with the stretcheded arms while bending the waist. Exhale at the same time. (Fig. 63)

c. When both hands reach the farthest end in the lower back, straighten the waist and lift up the arms. Make arched lines with both hands at the sides of the body and stretch the arms above the head with the palms forward. Inhale at the same time.

2) Essentials

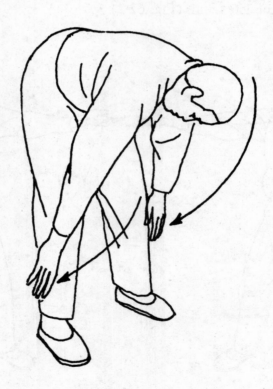

Fig. 63

It is important to stretch the arms straight. Inhale when bending the waist and exhale when stretching it.

Exercise ten times.

7. Supporting a Ball in Front of the Shoulder

1) Exercise method

a. Bend the waist. When the hands reaching the farthest ends at lower back, stretch the waist without moving the left hand. Turn the right palm and raise it to left up. When the right hand reaches the height of the right shoulder, do the movement of supporting a ball and put the weight of the body on the left foot. Let the tiptoes of the right foot touch the ground. Exhale at the same time. Then return the right hand to the lower right side. (Fig. 64-1)

b. Shift the weight of the body to the right foot. Let the tiptoe of the left foot touch the ground at the same time turn the left palm and lift it to the upper right from the lower left. When the left hand reaches the height of the left shoulder, do the movement of supporting a ball and exhale. Then return the left hand to the lower left. (Fig. 64-2)

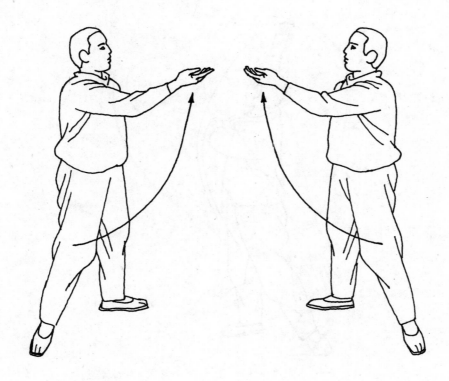

Fig. 64-1　　　　　　　　　　Fig. 64-2

2) Essential

When "supporting" a ball with the hands, the eyes look at the place where the "ball" is being supported and press the ground firmly with the tip of the foot of the same side. Coordinate the movements of supporting a ball, pressing the ground and breathing.

8. Turning the Body to Gaze at the Moon

1)Exercise method

Stand naturally. Wave both hands to the upper left and at the same time turn the upper part of the body to the left and turn the head left back. When waving both hands to the upper right, turn the upper part of the body to the right and raise the head up right as though looking at the moon. Inhale at the same time. Then return to the natural standing posture and exhale. (Fig. 65)

2) Essentials

The movements of waving the hands and turning the waist and head should be coordinated and reach the high level.

9. Turning the Waist and Pushing the Palms

1) Exercise method

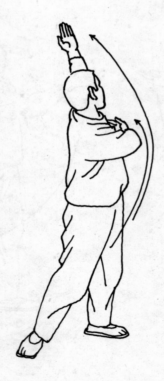

Fig. 65

a. Stand in the horse riding stance. Clench both hands and let them hang akimbo with the fist centres up and the tiger's mouth facing out. Draw the left elbow backward, turn the upper part of the body to the left, straighten right hand and push it out with strength. Inhale at the same time. Then return the original posture and exhale. (Fig. 66-1).

b. Draw the right elbow back, turn the upper part of the body to the right, change the left fist into a palm and push it out. Inhale at the same time. (Fig. 66-2)

2) Essentials

Pushing the palm forward is the movement of stretching the wrist with the fingers up and the hypothenar facing forward. Push one hand forward while drawing back the other. The strength is putting forth to the opposite sides. Inhale when pushing rightwards and exhale when pushing leftwards.

10. Horse Riding Stance with Hands Moving Like Clouds

1) Exercise method

a. Push the left hand out, with the palm inward at the level of the eyes and move the right hand forward with its palm facing the left at the level of the navel.

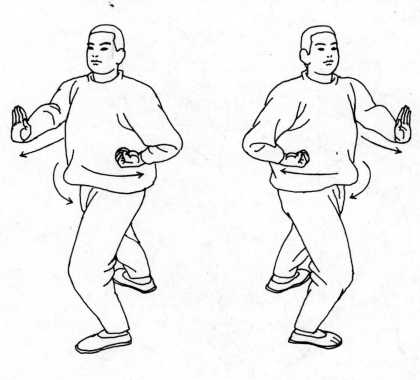

Fig. 66-1   Fig. 66-2

Turn the waist to the left while moving both hands left along. Inhale at the same time. (Fig. 67-1)

b. Turn the waist to the left as far as you can, while lifting the right hand to the height of the eye with the palm facing inward and bring down the left hand to the level of the navel with the palm facing the right. Move both hands to the right along with the turning of the waist. Exhale at the same time. (Fig. 67-2)

2) Essentials

The movements of the hands should be gentle. The eyes always follow the upper hand.

11. Dredging the Sea and Looking at the Sky

1) Exercise method

a. Stand in the left bow stance. Bend the upper part of the body forward, cross the hands in front of the left knee, and inhale at the same time. (Fig. 68-1)

b. Lift the crossed hands upward while leaning back the upper part of the body. Separate the hands after they have passed the top of the head with palms then facing each other. Raise the head to look at the sky and exhale at the same time. Bend the upper part of the body forward, press down both hands and cross them in front of the knees. Repeat the above movements. (Fig. 68-2)

2) Essentials

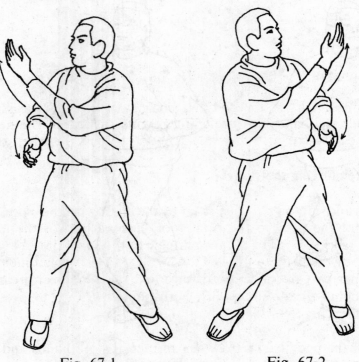

Fig. 67-1   Fig. 67-2

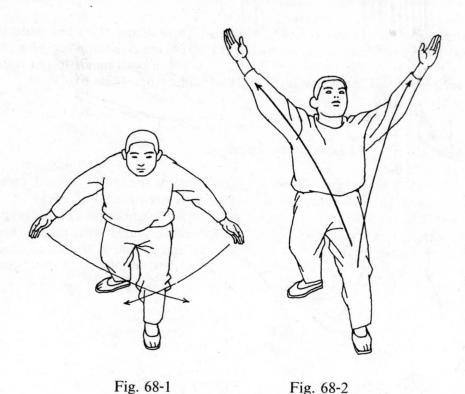

Fig. 68-1   Fig. 68-2

Inhale when the upper part of the body is bending forward and crossing the hands, and exhale when the hands are stretching beyond the top of the head and eyes are looking at the sky. Stretch the hands as much as possible when the eyes are looking at the sky.

12. Pushing and Reinforcing the Waves

1) Exercise method

a. Bend the elbows and put the hands in front of the chest with the palms facing out. Shift the weight of the body to the right foot. Let the heel of the left foot touch the ground and raise the tips of the toes. Inhale at the same time. (Fig. 69-1)

b. Shift the weight of the body to the left foot with its whole sole touching the ground. Move the upper part of the body forward and raise the heel of the right foot, with its tip touching the ground. Push both hands forward at eye-height. Exhale at the same time. (Fig. 69-2)

2) Essentials

Shift the weight of the body backward when retracting both hands and exhale at the same time. The movements should be done like the surging waves and

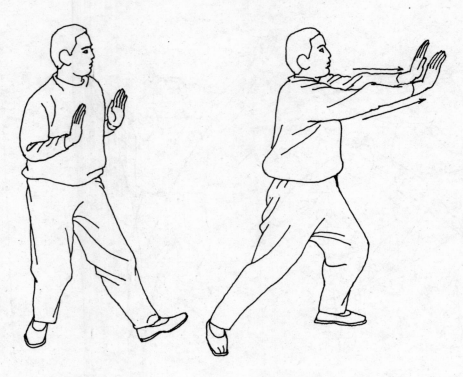

Fig. 69-1   Fig. 69-2

billows of the sea.

13. Flying Pigeon Spreading its Wings

1) Exercise method

a. Straighten the arms and turn the palms facing each other. Shift the weight of the body to the right foot, raise the tiptoe of the left foot, and inhale at the same time. (Fig. 70-1)

b. Spread the hands to the sides of the body horizontally as much as possible. Shift the weight of the body to the left foot, raise the heel of the right foot and exhale at the same time. (Fig. 70-2)

2) Essentials

When leaning back, spread both hands as though a flying pigeon were spreading its wings. The movements should be done in harmony with breathing.

14. Stretching the Arms While Charging the Fist

1) Exercise method:

Change the bow stance into the horse riding stance. Clench the hands and put them on the both sides of the waist with the centres facing up.

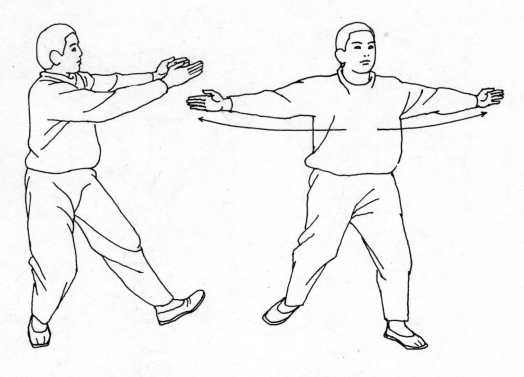

Fig. 70-1   Fig. 70-2

a. Push forward the right fist first and inhale. Then pull it back to the side of the waist and exhale. (Fig. 71-1)

b. Push forward the left fist and inhale. Pull it back to the side of waist and exhale. (Fig. 71-2)

2) Essentials

When changing from the bow stance to the horse riding stance, exhale somewhat softly and long. Breathe shortly and quickly when changing the fist and keep the eyes looking at the fist.

15. The Flying Wild Goose

1) Exercise method

a. Stand with both hands lifted up horizontally at the sides of the body with the feet a shoulder width apart.

b. Squat down as low as possible. Press both hands down as though a wild goose were flying. Exhale at the same time. (Fig. 72-1)

c. Stand up and lift both hands up. Inhale at the same time. (Fig. 72-2)

2) Essentials

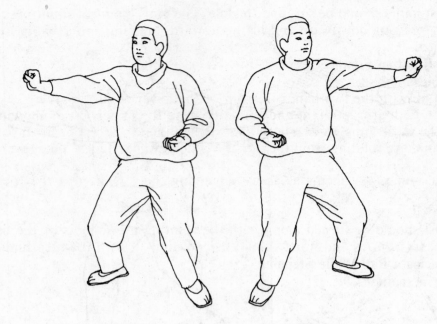

Fig. 71-1   Fig. 71-2

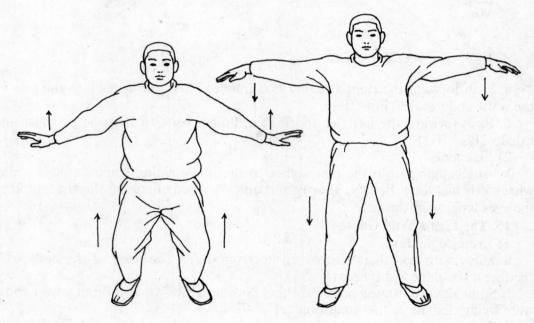

Fig. 72-1   Fig. 72-2

The wrist joints should be soft and flexible. The movements of squatting down, standing up, pressing downward and lifting upward, inhaling and exhaling should be coordinated.

16. The Rotating Flywheel
1) Exercise method

a. Stand up with the two hands in front of the lower belly.

b. Stretch both arms straight and rotate them to the upper left along with the turning of the waist. Inhale when both hands reach the top of the head and exhale when the hands are rotating from the upper left downward. Repeat the movements ten times.(Fig. 73-1)

c. Do the same movements as above, changing the direction of the rotation. (Fig. 73-2)

2) Essentials

The waist should be turned along with the rotating movements of the hands. The movements of arms and waist should be coordinated with the breathing.

17. Bouncing a Ball While Stepping
1) Exercise method

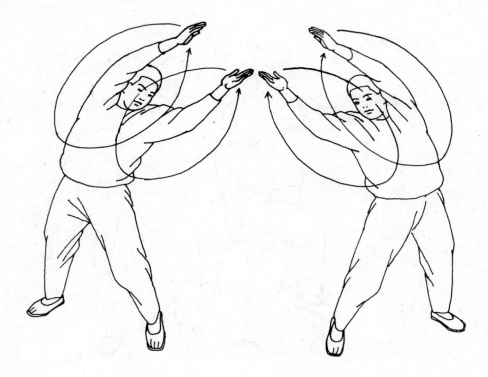

Fig. 73-1   Fig. 73-2

a. Lift up the left leg, do the movements of bouncing a ball with the right hand in front of the right shoulder. Inhale at the same time. (Fig. 74)

b. Lift up the right leg, do the movements of bouncing a ball with the left hand in front of the left shoulder. Exhale at the same time.

2) Essentials

The movements of lifting hand, bouncing the ball and stepping feet should be coordinated with breathing, and the stepping movements should be done in a very happy and relaxed manner.

Doing bouncing movements with the right and left hand once each is considered one sequence. Exercise ten times.

18. Pressing the Palms and Regulating the Breath

1) Exercise method

a. Stand with both hands in front of the lower belly.

b. Let the palms face up and lift them up to the front of eyes. Inhale at the same time. (Fig. 75-1)

c. Turn the palms with the fingers pointing at each other. Press them down from the front of eyes to the front of the lower belly. Exhale at the same time. (Fig. 75-2)

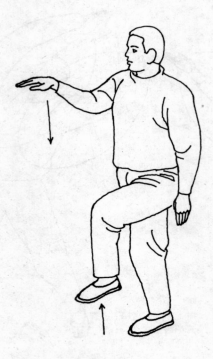

Fig. 74

2) Essentials

Inhale when lifting the hands up and exhale when pressing them down. The movements should be done slowly. One lifting and one pressing is considered one sequence. Exercise ten times.

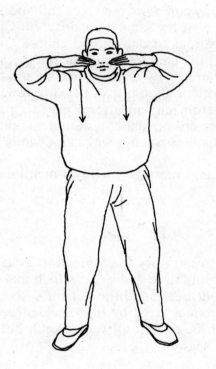
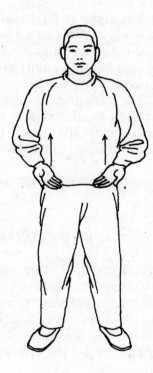

Fig. 75-1   Fig. 75-2

Chapter Three
QIGONG THERAPY FOR SOME COMMON DISEASES AND SERIOUS DISEASES

Qigong not only has curative effect on many common and frequently-occuring diseases, but also on some complicated diseases. At the same time, different Qigong exercises have different functions and effects, and so one should choose Qigong therapy according to his health condition and the characteristics of the disease in order for best results. In addition, during treatment by Qigong, one should avoid debilitating factors. For example, an ulcer patient should avoid taking raw, cold and pungent food which would irritate the stomach; an arteriosclerosis patient should avoid taking fatty foods; and a hypertension patient should maintain a healthy mood and avoid being over excited. Only in such a way can Qigong have its best effects.

(See Chapter Five for the point-pressing and massage methods mentioned in this chapter).

THE COMMON COLD

The common cold, also called acute upper respiratory tract infection, is usually caused by exposure to cold and wetness, and being tired and weak, which make the defensive mechanism of the respiratory tract decrease and the patient susceptible to bacteria and virus. The common cold is characterized by high incidence, high infectiousness and more complications. It can be caught all year round, but it is seen more in winter and spring than in other seasons.

1. Clinical Manifestations

The main symptoms of the common cold are headaches, stuffy nose, running nose, sneezing, chills and fever, etc.

2. Qigong Treatment

1) Quiescent Sitting Health Cultivation Exercise

Practise 1 to 2 times a day, 30 to 60 minutes each time. see Chapter Two for details.

2) Relaxed and Quiescent Recumbent Exercise

Practise 1 to 2 times a day, 30 to 60 minutes each time. See Chapter Two for details.

3) Health Cultivation Massage

Choose combing the hair, dry-washing the face, knocking the ears, tapping the teeth, rocking the limbs, rubbing the foot's arch and dry bath and practise several times a day.

4) Conducting and Leading Exercise

Rub the palms till warm, massage the Fengfu point for about 100 times. Then cross the hands to hold the opposite Fengfu points tightly, bow forward for about 100 times and concentrate the mind on Qihai point for 10 to 15 minutes. It is necessary to keep a peaceful and stable mood and natural respiration.

5) Slight-perspiratory Exercise

Take the standing posture. Raise the left hand with the palm upward and push it with force. At the same time stamp the left foot. Inhale with the nose, exhale with the mouth. Repeat the above movement for 40 times until the whole body perspires slightly. If not perspiring, do the same movements with right hand 40 times again.

6) Expectant Point Massage

Press and massage different points according to the different types of cold, such as cold-wind, hot-wind, poor constitution, etc. Usually press and knead the following points: Fengfu, Fengchi, Hegu, Yingxiang, Dazhui, Shaoshang, Taiyang, Zusanli, and Lieque points and make them gain *qi*.

3. Sample Case

Ms. Zhu, 28 years old, was very weak and often suffered from cold at the change of seasons and alternating cold and hot weather, often accompanied with headaches, dizzy, stuffy nose, sore throat, cough, tiredness, weakness, and anepithymia. Only after taking medicine did she feel a little better. Last spring, she caught a cold again, and began to practise Qigong, meanwhile taking some medicine. After one week, she recovered. She has been practising Qigong since then. Now she is in good health and has not caught a cold since.

NEURASTHENIA

Neurasthenia (or neurosism) is a kind of common functional disease, resulting from disorders of cerebral function caused by over-tiredness, worry, over-strain and depression. It often appears in mental workers and young and middle-aged people.

1. Clinical Manifestations

The patient is easily excited or depressed and experiences accompanying headaches, giddiness, insomnia, hypomnesis, distractibility, restlessness, irritability unstable moods, anxiety or depression. Most patients cannot sleep well, are liable to wake up, have vivid dreams or even can not sleep at all at night. They may also have the following symptoms: maldigestion, distention, constipation, anorexia and irregular menstruation in women, impotence and seminal emission in men, etc.

2. Qigong Treatment

1) Relaxed and Quiescent Recumbent Exercise

Relax and get into quiescent naturally, and concentrate the mind on Dantian. Make the breathing deep, long, even, gentle, and slow, so as to combine the original *qi* inside the body with the air outside, and refine them into the internal *qi* to circulate all over the body. Practise 2 to 3 times a day. See Chapter Two for the details.

2) Rocking Exercise

This exercise has the function of removing the nervous messages in the mind and treating insomnia. Sit on the bed with the legs naturally bent and crossed before going to bed. First, massage the Shenyu and Mingmen points on the waist with the palms for 36 times, then massage Yongquan point in the centre of the left and right soles with the palms for 36 times each, so as to keep the mind in quiescence and the spirit stable. Then sit peacefully for a moment, close the eyes slightly, concentrate the mind and breathe calmly, lick the palate, and put the hands on the knees. Taking the waist as the axis, rock the upper body in a circle for 36 times to the right and another 36 times to the left. The rocking should be from small to large and while rocking, the head and neck should swing to and fro in correspondence with the body. Concentrate the mind and breath on Dantian. Practise 1 to 2 times a day.

3) Relaxed and Tense Sleep-promoting Exercise

This is a set of exercises designed first to tense the muscles and then relax them. It helps the neurosism patient to go to sleep. Practise before going to bed. The method is as follows:

a. Stand naturally with the arms hanging down. Then raise the arms forward to the shoulder level, clench the hands, and make the muscles of upper arms tense, inhaling at the same time. Then bend the upper body slightly, hang down the arms and swing them to and fro, to make the muscles of the upper arms and shoulder joints relax fully, recite the word relax silently, exhaling at the same time. Repeat 6 to 9 times.

b. The starting posture is the same as the one in part (a). Bend the elbows of the arms, and raise them to the shoulder level, clench the hands, put the fists in front of the chest, contract the muscles of the shoulders and upper arms with force, exhaling at the same time. Hang down the arms, bend the upper body forward slightly, relax the mind, the shoulders and elbows fully, exhaling at the same time. Repeat 6 to 9 times.

c. Stand with the feet close together and the arms hanging down in front of the body, with the fingers interlocked. Then lift the heels, raise the arms upward and contract the muscles all over the body with force, inhaling at the same time. Then lower down the arms, move the two hands apart, squat down and bend the head forward naturally to make the muscles all over the body fully relaxed, exhaling at the same time. Repeat 6 to 9 times.

d. Take the sitting posture. Interlock the hands and put them on the back of the head, then throw the head backward with force while pulling the two hands forward against the head and opening the lower jaw slightly to make the muscles of the head and the neck tense, inhaling at the same time. Then relax the head, neck and hands, exhaling at the same time. Repeat 6 to 9 times.

e. Take the sitting posture. Put the hands on the knees, then press the hands on the thighs, stamp the ground with the feet forcefully to make the muscles of the lower limbs tense, inhaling at the same time. Then relax the mind and the lower and upper limbs fully, exhaling at the same time. Repeat 6 to 9 times.

f. Take the supine lying posture. Place the arms at the two sides of the body with the palms pressing downward and the back and the waist slightly stiff to make the muscles of the back and the waist tense, inhaling at the same time. Then relax the arms and the mind, the back and the waist, exhaling at the same time. Repeat 6 times.

g. Take the supine lying posture. Interlock the fingers and put the hands on the back of the head. Raise the head slightly and contract the muscles of the lower abdomen. Then lower the head, and relax the muscles of the lower abdomen meanwhile putting the hands on the abdomen one above the other, massaging clockwise and reciting the word relax silently. Repeat 3 to 5 times.

h. Lying on your side. Put the arms in front of the head with the elbows bent at about 90 degrees. Put the two legs one on the other, bend the knees at about 120 degrees, put the upper foot behind the lower one, and close the eyes. Then contract the muscles of the fingers and toes and inhale at the same time. Exhale when relaxing and reciting silently, "It is wonderful to relax. I feel extremely comfortable and I even would not move my fingers and toes."

i. The beginning posture is the same as in part (h). Recite silently "relax, I feel very comfortable." Relax gradually all the muscles and put the mind in a quiescent state.

4) Standing Straight Like a Stake Cultivation Exercise

Take the natural standing posture. Practise twice a day. See Chapter Two for details.

5) Expectant Point Massage

This is used to treat neurosism patients who have the following symptoms: headaches, insomnia and weakness of the body.

a. Press the Zanzhu, Yangbai, Shangxing, Baihui, Taiyang, Fengchi and Yintang points.

b. Press and knead the Ermen and Tinggong points.

c. Knead the auricles and pull the earlobes.

d. Press and knead the Zusanli and Sanyinjiao points.

Repeat the above point-pressing massage 9 to 18 times for each.

In short, neurosism patients should practise both quiescent and motional exercise according to their own constitution and state of health.

3. Sample Case

Mr.Chen, 55 years old, had suffered from dizzy, headaches, and insomnia for many years, and had suffered from short breath, palpitation, failing memory and had a low work efficiency for more than ten years. He was diagnosed as having neurasthenia and treated with a combination of Western and tradtional Chinese medicine, but there was no obvious and stable effect. Then he turned to Qigong treatment. After practising for two weeks, the insomnia and headaches were relieved. Two months later, the above symptoms disappeared and he gained weight, experienced an increase in appetite, and his mental and physical condition and memory were also improved. Now he can perform his normal responsibilities well.

INSOMNIA

Insomnia is when the patient cannot fall asleep normally.

1. Clinical Manifestations

The patients who do not have serious insomnia find it difficult to fall asleep, or sleep lightly, dream and wake up frequently and cannot sleep again. The serious cases cannot sleep for one or several nights, accompanied with dizziness, slow reactions and a reduction of intelligence.

2. Qigong Treatment

1) Hypnotic exercise

Exercise your limbs before practice. Then in bed, press Baihui point in the middle of the top of your head and Taiyang point in the sides of your head separately. Impress the positions of these points in your mind. Then lie down in a comfortable positure. Do not put your hands on the chest. Relax yourself and breathe freely. When exhaling, concentrate your mind on driving the *qi* up to Baihui and Taiyang. When inhaling, move the *qi* down to Dantian. At the same time, think to yourself "I have relaxed. I am going to sleep." Get rid of disturbances, make yourself relaxed, happy, carefree and joyous and gradually fall asleep.

2) Quiescent Relaxing and Tensing Exercise

Close your eyes lightly and lie on your back. Bend your knees at an angle of 145 degrees. In this way, you can concentrate your mind on the lower limbs. When the original disturbance is dismissed from your mind and you feel a little tired, stretch one of the two lower limbs but keep the other one bending and exchange the posture of the two lower limbs. After a few minutes, the two lower limbs will be stretched and relaxed. Or you can also keep them bent until you almost fall asleep and then stretch the legs naturally. It is normal for you to feel your lower limbs rocking and find difficulty in standing when you are near to sleeping.

3) Breath Listening and Counting Method

Listen to the sound of your respiration and count it out simply, "one, two, three," "one, two, three," begining again each fourth breath. Practise this until you cannot count clearly or cannot hear clearly.

4) Refer to the exercises in the previous section of neurasthenia.

3. Sample Case

Mr. He had suffered insomnia for about ten years and could fall asleep only after taking sleeping pills. Otherwise, he would not be able to fall asleep and would feel dizzy and dazed and experience headaches. Through practising Qigong, he recovered dramatically and could sleep about 6 hours every night.

CHRONIC BRONCHITIS AND EMPHYSEMA

Chronic bronchitis is a kind of common disease in middle-aged and old people, especially in the cold seasons and regions. And it can develop into a complication called emphysema.

1. Clinical Manifestations

The main symptoms are chronic and recurrent coughing, accompanied with sputum and gasping and occurring according to the seasons, especially in winter. After recurring without being cured, it may develop into emphysema and the patient may have short breath, especially after activity and have a lot of white and thick sputum. Breathing will become difficult and the face of the patient will turn to red and blue.

2. Qigong Treatment

1) Quiescent Sitting Health Cultivation Exercise

Usually, practise in the way of breathing naturally or using the second respiration method, 30 minutes at a time, 4 to 6 times a day. See Chapter Two for details.

2) Relaxed and Quiescent Recumbent Exercise

Practise 30 minutes at a time, 3 to 4 times a day. See Chapter Two for further details.

3) *Qi* Reinforcing Exercise

a. Long exhaling. Stand straight naturally, relax the muscles and exhale deeply and fully through the nose. After exhaling the air completely, inhale naturally and imagine that the *qi* goes to the lower abdomen. Make the exhale longer than the inhale, with time ratio of from 3:2 to 2:1, limiting this to a degree at which you don't feel dizzy. Repeat 10 to 30 times.

b. Natural breathing. Standing naturally and breathe naturally for about 30 seconds.

c. Breathing with bound chest. Stand naturally. Cross the arms in front of the chest and press your chest to exhale. Then, slowly raise the two arms to relieve the pressure of the chest and inhale. The main points to the breath is the same as in section (a). Repeat 10 to 30 times.

d. Natural breathing. Stand naturally. Swing the two arms left and right freely and breathe naturally for 30 seconds.

e. Bending the waist while exhaling. Stand naturally. Cross the two arms in front of the abdomen and exhale when bending forward. Return to the beginning posture. Then inhale with the two arms stretched to the two sides. The main points for breathing is the same as in section (a). Repeat 10 to 30 times.

f. Chest-pressed exhaling. Stand naturally. Press the two hands on the chest. Exhale when pressing the chest, and inhale when returnning to the beginning state. The main points for breathing is the same as in section (a). Repeat 10 to 30 times.

g. Breathing naturally: Same as in section (d).

h. Breathing by holding the knees. Stand naturally. Raise one leg, hold the knee with your hands to press the abdomen tightly and exhale. Then inhale when returning to the beginning state. The main points for the breathing is the same as in section (a). Repeat 10 to 30 times.

i. Blowing method

Sit or stand. Hang a cotton ball at the mouth level and half metre away from the mouth. Blow the ball slowly and keep blowing as long as you can until the breath runs out. After inhaling naturally, blow it again. Repeat 10 times.

j. Turning the body and tapping the chest.

Stand, with arms hanging down naturally. Tap the chest while turning the body to the left then the right, keeping the muscles relaxed and breathing naturally. Repeat 30 times.

4) Three 8-Shape *Qi* Driving Cultivation Exercise

a. Take the sitting posture. Relax and calm yourself. Stretch the hands with the palms down and put them on the lap. Clench the left or the right hand into a fist with the palm forward. Put the joint of the index finger on Shangen point and move the fist around the two eye rims from this point, as if writing the number 8 around the eye rims, first clockwise and then counter clockwise each for 50 to 100 times. Breathe once for every 8. Then use the other hand to do it. While doing this, clench the other hand into half fist and put it on the lap with its palm down. (Figs. 76-1, 2)

b. The posture is the same as in (a). Clench the hand into a fist with the palm forward. Put the joint of the index finger on Renzhong point. Move the fist around the mouth from this point and when the fist comes back to the point, make another circle along the outside line of one eye, across the forehead, then downward along the outside of the other eye until back to Renzhong. Write this 8 clockwise and counter clockwise 50 to 100 times each. Breathe once for every 8. Change to the other hand, repeating this 1-2 times. (Fig. 76-3)

c. Clench a hand with the palm forward. Put the joint of the index finger on the supertemporal arteria before one ear, move the fist in a circle around the helix and back to the original position. Then move it down to the lower jaw, along the outline of this side of the face, up to the forehead and back to the beginning point. Breathe once for every 8. Write this 8 clockwise and counter clockwise 50 to 100 times each. Do it on the both sides of the face 1-2 times each. The suitable rate is 5-8 circles per minute. Practise 30 minutes each time, 2-3 times every day. (Fig.76-4)

5) Longevity Exercise

Choose the 6th, 7th, 8th, 11th and 21th sections to practise. See Chapter Two for the specific methods.

6) Expectant Point Massage

Knead the Taiyang, Fengchi, Tiantu and Dazhui points with the thumb or index finger. Repeat 20 times. Then hit the back opposite the lower chest with the fists and tap the chest with the palms.

Patients ought to choose the above exercises according to their illness. When the patient is seriouslly ill and finds it difficult to stand up, it would be better to practise the Quiescent Sitting Health Cultivation Exercise and the Relaxed and

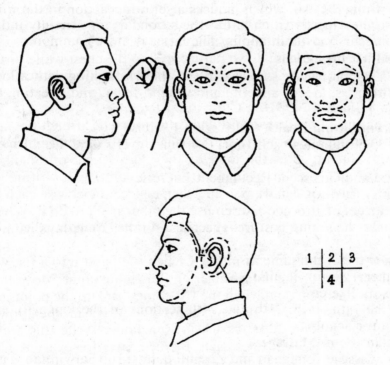

Figs. 76-1, 2, 3, 4

Quiescent Recumbent Exercise, and breathe naturally. When the health condition becomes better, the patient can practise *Qi* Reinforcing Exercise and the others.

3. Sample Case

Mr. Wu, 63 years old, had suffered from chronic coughing for about 20 years and gasping for about 10 years. He had serious gasping with a lot of sputum and found it difficult to lie on a bed and felt distressed in the chest when walking in the room.

After 3 months of practising Qigong, the symptoms were relieved and the patient was able to go up and down the stairs to the second floor. It was found that his lung capacity had increased by 50 percent through inspection and the tidal volume was increased from 416 to 784 ml. The ECG inspection before the Qigong treatment showed that he had signs of cor pulmonale disease, but most of them were relieved after six months of Qigong exercises.

TUBERCULOSIS

Tuberculosis is a chronic infection and comsuptive disease caused by lung infections of mycotacterium tuberculosis. It is classified into primary and secondary. Primary tuberculosis, which induces a serious reaction in the whole body of the patient, occurs mostly in children; the secondary one mainly induces a local reaction and occurs mostly in adults. The latter is more common.

1. Clinical Manifestations

The main symptoms are soreness in the chest, coughing with a lot of sputum and blood, tiredness, loss of appetite and weight, fever, and sweating at night.

2. Qigong Treatment

1) Quiescent Sitting Health Cultivation Exercise

Practise 30-60 minutes each time, 3-4 times every day. See Chapter Two for details.

2) Relaxed and Quiescent Recumbent Exercise

See Chapter Two for details.

3) Eight Pieces of Brocade Exercise

Usually take the sitting posture. Practise 2-4 times each day. See Chapter Two for details.

4) Sinew-Transforming Exercise.

See Chapter Two for details.

5) Longevity Exercise

Practise the 14th, 16th, 21th and 24th sections of the longevity exercise. See Chapter Two for details.

6) Expectant Point Massage

Press and massage Tongguan and Zusanli points; rub Sanyinjiao, Yanglingquan and Yongquan points.

3. Sample Case

Mr. Ma, 49 years old, suffered from IV style lung tuberculosis, accompanied with spontaneous pneumothorax in the right lung. He was hospitalized because of haemoptysis, but had no response to the treatment with haemostatic and anti-tuberculosis medicine. After practising Qigong for half a year, the haemoptysis was stopped. One year later, his health condition was much better. The X-ray examination showed that the focus was absorbed and the hole was closed, and the sputum examination for tubercle bacillus showed positive reactions. He continued practising sitting and standing exercises coordinated with motional exercises and jogging. His constitution became healthy and strong gradually. He has had no relapse in the past ten years.

BRONCHIAL ASTHMA

Bronchial asthma is a kind of common allergic reaction disease of the bronchial tubes. People may suffer from this kind of disease at any age. It often attacks in autumn and winter. It is one of the allergic diseases.

1. Clinical Manifestations

Before the disease attacks, symptoms include itching in the nose, sneezing, itching in the throat, coughing and chest distress. It often attacks suddenly at night. The symptoms are chest distress, short breath, dyspnea, shortness of inhaling and prolonging of exhaling accompanied with wheezing, dysphoria and profuse sweating. When the disease gets severe, symptoms such as oxygen deficiency, pale face and cyanosis of the lips and fingers will appear. At the early stage, the patient has dry cough and thick sputum and finds it hard to breathe until the foam like sputum is spit. The symptoms may last several minutes, but in the most cases may last a half an hour, or even a few days.

2. Qigong Treatment

1) Quiescent Sitting Health Cultivation Exercise.

2) Relaxed and Quiescent Recumbent Exercise.

The above exercises can be used when the disease suddenly attacks. Do the Quiescent Sitting Health Cultivation Exercise mainly and the Relaxed and Quiescent Recumbent Exercise as the auxiliary one. Adopt the first and the second respiration methods alternately for the exercises. Practise 30 to 60 minutes at a time and 4 to 5 times a day. Meanwhile, rub Tian and Shanzhong points and the front chest with the palms successively for 36 times. See Chapter Two for details.

3) Wall-pushing Exercise

a. Concentrate the mind on Shanzhong. Breathe naturally and stand with feet a shoulder width. Put body against the wall at an angle of 15-20 degrees. Hold the ground with the toes of both feet firmly. Stand straight and raise the arms straight up or obliquely straight up. Put the palms on the wall. Raise the arms with force, but not too straight. Press the wall with your arms strongly and continously for five minutes.

b. Concentrate the mind on Shanzhong point. Breathe naturally, and stand with the feet a shoulder width. Put your body against the wall at an angle of 20-30 degrees. Hold the ground with your toes firmly. Contract your abdomen slightly. Stretch the arms to each side of the body. Put the palms on the wall and push the wall with force continuously for five minutes.

This method can be used during the period of acute attack. Practise it 3 times a day.

4) Longevity Exercise

Practise the 1st, 6th, 7th, 8th and 11th sections. Exercise 2 or 3 times a day. See Chapter two for details.

In brief, the patient should choose the above exercise reasonably according to the constitution and the condition of the disease.

3. Sample Case

Mr. Liu, 66 years old, had suffered from bronchial asthma for many years. In recent years, the disease attacked from time to time because of the change of the climate and his overwork. He spent most of his time in winter lying in bed and it was hard for him to lie flat.

After the treatment with both western and traditional Chinese medicine, his illness could not be controlled or relieved. Then he turned to Qigong treatment and began to practise Qigong. Relaxation, quiescence and breathing naturally were emphasized in his practice. A month later he experienced fewer asthma attacks. After 4 months, the symptoms had almost disappeared, and his appetite and condition of his health had improved. There have been no severe attacks in the past three years and he can now walk in the yard instead of lying in bed in winter.

PNEUMOSILICOSIS

Pneumosilicosis is a kind of disease of the respiratory system which damages the function of the lungs. This disease is caused by inspiring silicon dioxide-containing dust over a long time, after which the lung tissue becomes lungs-fibrosis. The majority of patients are workers who engage in mining, quarrying, asbestos manufacture, powder and glass making.

1. Clinical Manifestations

Main symptoms are dry coughing, tiredness, breathing difficulties when doing something with force, and catching cold easily. In the advanced stage, it may develop into emphysema and complication of pulmonary function. It is also possible to develop pneumothorax and tuberculosis at the same time.

2. Qigong Treatment

1) Quiescent Sitting Health Cultivation Exercise

Practise with the 1st and 2nd respiration methods alternately. Exercise 3 or 4 times a day and 30-60 minutes each time. See Chapter Two for details.

2) Relaxed and Quiescent Recumbent Exercise

Practise with the 1st and the 2nd respiration methods alterntely. Do it 3 or 4 times a day and 30-60 minutes each time. This exercise can be practised with the Quiescent Sitting Health Cultivation Exercise. See Chapter Two for details.

3) Morning Walking Exercise

See Chapter Two for the details.

4) Longevity Exercise

Select the 1st, 6th, 7th, 14th, 16th and 21st sections to practise. Exercise 3 or 4 times a day and 30 minutes each time. Refer to Chapter Two for the details.

5) Health Cultivation Massage

See Chapter Two for details. This method can be practised alternately with the Quiescent Sitting Health Cultivation Exercise.

6) Sinew-transforming Exercise

See Chapter Two for details.

7) *Qi* Recinforing Exercise

See the previous sections about the chronic bronchitis and emphysema of the lungs for details.

In brief, the patient should select the exercises according to the health condition and disease, and can do the above exercises alternately. Regardless of the exercise chosen, it should be persistently done step by step. It is also all right to do long-distance jogging, during which inhales and exhales should be taken once every four paces, and use the natural environment to do such exercises as sunbathing sun and air baths, water baths, and swimming in order to increase the vital capacity of the lungs.

3. Sample Case

Mr. Qian, 56 years old, had done work in which he was exposed to powdery air for over ten years. He suffered from chest pain, coughing, frequent colds for years. Light activity could lead him to have chest distress and rapid breathing. His physical strength had decreased obviously. X-ray examination showed that the hilus of his lung and his lung markings were not clear and there were some pneumosilicosis nodes.

After three months of Qigong exercise, his clinical manifestation improved obviously. X-ray re-examination showed that the clarity of his hilus pulmonis and his lung markings had improved significantly. His physical strength has increased and now he can do some light work.

BRONCHIECTASIC DISEASE

This disease is the development of long-term bronchitis with the surrounding fibrous tissus pulled, bronchis twisted and deformed, accumulating gases and sputum in distal trachea and increase of pressure within the bronchis.

1. Clinical Manifestation

Coughing repeatedly and spitting thick sputum and blood are the main symptoms. The course of the disease is comparatively long.

2. Qigong Treatment

1) Quiescent Sitting Health Cultivation Exercise

Adopt the natural breathing method or the second breathing method. Do the exercise 3 to 5 times a day, 30 minutes each time. See Chapter Two for details.

2) Relaxed and Quiescent Recumbent Exercise

See Chapter Two.

3) Eight Pieces of Brocade Exercise

Take the sitting posture. Do the exercise 2 to 4 times a day, 30 minutes each time.

4) Three 8-shape *Qi* Driving Cultivation Exercise

See the previous sections of chronic bronchitis and emphysema of the lungs.

PNEUMOTHORAX

Pneumothorax is a kind of disease caused by air entering into the thoracic cavity through a breach created when the visceral pleaura and alveoli of the lungs break up. The idiopathic and spontaneous pneumothorax refer to those patients who have no obvious clinical manifestation. The majority of the patients are young people. Some chronic disease of the lungs, such as chronic bronchitis, emphysema, asthma, tuberculosis and pulmonary fibrosis may be also accompanied with pneumothorax at the same time. This is common in old people.

1. Clinical Manifestation

Usually patients experience acute attacks with chest distress and later chest pains accompanied with an irritating cough, dyspnea, restlessness and even coma.

2. Qigong Treatment

1) Longevity Exercise

Do the exercises of some sections. See Chapter Two for details.

2) Six-word Respiration Exercise

The six words in Chinese are *hushui*—water of the lake, which means smoothness; *wufeng*—no wind, which means quiescence; and *xuri*—the rising sun, which means rising. The six-word formula is recited in order to direct the mind. Sit quietly with the legs crossed and the chest slightly pulling in. Put one hand on the other with Neilaogong point of the upper hand touching Wailaogong point of the lower hand. Don't think anything, stay in balance and breathe naturally. Let the body combine with the mind as one. Keep like this for a while, so that the circulation *qi* and blood will be stimulated. Practise it for no less than 60 minutes each time.

If the lung capacity compression is more than 20 percent of normal or pneumothorax has existed for over three days, the patient should be sent to the hospital to be treated with traracic manometry and air extraction. Qigong exercise can be considered as a kind of auxiliary means of treatment. If the lung compression is less than 20 percent and there are no symptoms such as dyspnea and chest pain, Qigong can be used as the main means of the treatment.

3. Sample Case

Mr. Sun, married, 37 years old, is a foundry man. He went to hospital to have acupuncture for a backache. When the therapy was over, he felt dyspnea and shortness of breath. The dyspnea increased that night and he could not lie down because of the backache. The illness was diagnosed as pneumothorax after examination. He turned to Qigong treatment, practising the longevity and the Mashan (horse-hill) exercises as the main treatment while taking orally compound tablets of liquorice as an auxiliary means. After Qigong exercises and taking the medicine following the doctor's advice, he could lie down that very night and the pain was alleviated. After three days, he could walk and do some house work. The X-ray examination showed that the lung compression was 30 percent. Seven days later, he could grow vegetables.

VIRUS PNEUMONIA

Virus pneumonia is a kind of inflammation of lungs caused by influenza virus, myxovirus, measles, chicken pox, herpes zoster virus, etc. It often appears in spring and winter.

1. Clinical Manifestation

The main symptoms are headache, a lack of strength, fever, coughing, spitting thick sputum, as well as continuous high fever, palpitation, shortness of breath, cyanosis, etc.

2. Qigong Treatment

1) Quiescent Sitting Health Cultivation Exercise

Adopt the first respiration method, and recite "the pneumonia will be cured" silently. Practise 3 to 6 times a day, 30 to 60 minutes each time. See Chapter Two.

2) Relaxed and Quiescent Recumbent Exercise

Adopt the first respiration method. Practise 3 times a day, 30 minutes each time. See Chapter Two.

3) Taiji Qigong

Practise 1 or 2 times a day, 30 minutes each time. See Chapter Two.

4) Six-word Respiration Exercise

Practise once a day. See previous section on pneumathorax.

3. Sample Case

Mr. Xu had suffered from virus pneumonia and occasionally allergic rhinitis, accompanied with weakness, anorexia, headache, coughing and palpitation, and did not recover after treatment with Western and traditional Chinese medicine. Then he turned to Qigong treatment, practising the Relaxed and Quiescent Recumbent Exercise. Half a month later, the sharp pain in his chest disappeared, his appetite increased and his general health got better. A month later, his condition improved further. He recovered completely before long.

CHRONIC GASTRITIS

Chronic gastritis is a kind of chronic inflammation of gastric mucosa. Usually, it can be divided into superficial gastritis, atrophic gastritis and hypertrophic gastritis.

1. Clinical Manifestations

The general manifestation of superficial gastritis is the discomfort, the sense of pressure and distension in the upper abdomen after eating, relieved after belching, sometimes accompanied with nausea, vomiting, vomiting acid and occasionally stomachache. It often occurs in men at age 20 to 40. The main symptoms of atrophic gastritis are anorexia, a bloated sensation after meals, dull pain in the upper abdomen and anaemia, loss of weight and tiredness. It often occurs in people over 40. Stubborn pain in the upper abdomen is the main symptom of the hypertrophic gastritis. Food and alkaline drugs can relieve the pain, which is similar to gastric and duodenal ulcer. But the pain is irregular and often accompanied with a sense of hunger and vomiting of acid.

2. Qigong Treatment

1) Quiescent Sitting Health Cultivation Exercise

This can reduce the gastric secretion and has an adjusting effect. The patient of hypertrophic gastritis should choose to practise it as the main means, with the Relaxed and Quiescent Recumbent Exercise as the auxiliary means. The patient should also practise it relatively often. Use the first respiration method. See Chapter Two for details.

2) Relaxed and Quiescent Recumbent Exercise

This exercise can increase gastric peristalsis and help to relieve the symptoms and realize the purpose of treatment. The patient of atrophic gastritis should use the second respiration method and practise the Quiescent Sitting Health Cultivation Exercise as the main means and a little Relaxed and Quiescent Recumbent Cultivation Exercise as the auxiliary means.

3) Taiji Qigong

See Chapter Two.

4) Three 8-Shape *Qi*-Driving Cultivation Exercise

See the previous sections on chronic bronchitis and emphysema.

5) Health Cultivation Massage

Choose tapping the teeth, swallowing and rubbing belly methods. Practise 4 to 6 times a day. See Chapter Two.

6) Longevity Exercise

See Chapter Two.

Qigong treatment has a peculiar effect on chronic gastritis. In particular the Quiescent Sitting Health Cultivation and Relaxed and Quiescent Recumbent Exercises can have a satisfactory effect for the patient, no matter what type of gastritis is being suffered, it is necessary to keep practising 2 to 4 times a day, 30 to 60 minutes each time. Also to avoid hot, cold and hot foods while practising Qigong exercises and eat food slowly in order to sustain the treatment.

3. Sample Case

Mr. Lu, 52 years old, had suffered from anorexia, slight pain and abdominal distension in the upper abdomen, tiredness and loss of weight for two years. The gastroscope examination showed that the mucosa of the stomach was low, the blood vessels under the gastric mucosa were clear and with the shape of a tree or a net, and the colour of the mucosa was pale. He was diagnosed as having chronic atrophic gastritis. His health condition did not improve after treatment with western and traditional Chinese medicine. So he turned to Qigong treatment. Half a month later, the abdominal distension and slight pain were relieved, and his appetite increased. Three months later, the accompanying symptoms had disappeared almost completely. He could eat more and gained weight. After six months, a gastroscope examination showed nothing abnormal in the stomach.

GASTRIC AND DUODENAL ULCER

Gastric and duodenal ulcer is a kind of chronic ulcer and systemic disease occurring in the stomach and duodenum. The incidence rate is about 10 percent among the population being particularly common in young and middle-aged adults.

1. Clinical Manifestations

The predominant symptoms are regular pain and distension in the lower abdomen, vomiting of acid, bowel sounds, and vomiting. The patient with a gastric ulcer usually feels pain in the stomach from half an hour to an hour after meals. The patient with duodenal ulcer usually feels pain when the stomach is empty, with the pain being relieved after meals.

2. Qigong Treatment

1) Quiescent Sitting Health Cultivation Exercise

See Chapter Two for details.

2) Relaxed and Quiescent Recumbent Exercise

Generally speaking, the people with comparatively better health condition should primarily practise the Quiescent Sitting Health Cultivation Exercise and take the Relaxed and Quiescent Recumbent Exercise as the auxiliary means, and vice versa for those who are weak. With the improvement of the health condition, the Quiescent Sitting Health Cultivation Exercise should be gradually practised as the main means. The patient with a good appetite but vomiting of acid should take the first respiration method. And those who have suffered from ulcer for a long time, and have the symptoms of anorexia, weakness, and abdominal distension, should take the second one. Practise 3 to 6 times a day, 30 to 60 minutes each time. See Chapter Two for details.

3) Longevity Exercise

Choose the 1st, 10th, 13th, 17th, and 29th sections. Practise 2 to 3 times a day, 30 minutes each time. See Chapter Two.

4) Health Cultivation Massage

Choose tapping the teeth, swallowing, and rubbing the belly methods. Practise 4 to 6 times a day. See Chapter Two.

5) Expectant Point Massage

Press Hegu, Zusanli, Neiguan and Shenmen each for several minutes to make them gain *qi*.

6) Other exercises

In order to improve the physical constitution and help to strengthen the effect of the treatment, Taiji Qigong and Standing Straight Like a Stake Exercise can also be practised at the same time. During the Qigong treatment, it is necessary for the patient to persist in practising. In addition, they should adjust their diet, avoid raw, cold, hard, hot food; eat more often each day but with less food each time, and keep the life regular and the mind pleasant. Cigarette and wine are forbidden. These will help the patient practise Qigong well, help the gastroenteric function recover and strengthen the effect of the treatment.

3. Sample Case

Mr. Zhang, 61 years old, had suffered from pain and discomfort in the upper abdomen for four years. The pain usually occurred when the stomach was empty and could be relieved after the expectant treatment. The pain became severe in October 1982, and he was diagnosed as having duodenal ulcer through X-ray barium meal examination and gastroscope (the ulcer was 2.5x2.0 cm). The expectant treatment had no obvious effect and he defecated tarry stool for three days in December the same year. He was hospitalized for three months, but the symptoms could not be relieved. The occult blood examination showed +++, and the reexamination by gastroscope showed that the ulcerated surface had not improved. Because the patient was afraid of operation, comprehensive Qigong treatment was adopted. While accepting expectant treatment of hemostasis, he began to practise Qigong. One week later, the pain was apparently relieved and the appetite had increased. Two months later, the clinical symptoms disappeared.

Reexamination by gastroscope showed that the ulcer had mostly healed. He persisted in the Qigong exercises after being discharged from the hospital. So far the effect is still stable.

GASTROPTOSIA

Gastroptosia refers to the position of the stomach being lower than normal. It is common in old people, especially in those who are weak.

1. Clinical Manifestations

The main symptoms are abdominal distension, pain in the upper abdomen, anorexia, indigestion, constipation, etc.

2. Qigong Treatment

1) Relaxed and Quiescent Recumbent Exercise

Lie on the back with a high pillow and put the palms on the bed. Put something under the buttocks so as to lift them 5 cm higher than the bed. Use the second respiration method and concentrate the mind on Dantian. Practise the exercise immediately after each meal, practising 30 to 60 minutes each time. See Chapter Two for details.

2) Heaven and Earth Exercise

Stand with the feet a shoulder width apart, half close the eyes, close the mouth lightly and relax. Hang the arms down at the waist, then raise them slowly above the head with the palms up. Cross the fingers and turn the palms. Meanwhile lift the heels and look at the sky, inhaling at the same time. Then squat slowly, moving the hands down along the sides of the body. Put the elbows close to the knees and the heels flat on the ground, exhaling at the same time. Repeat 10 to 20 times. Practise 4 to 6 times a day.

3) Qiaoqiao (Seesaw) Exercise

Lie on the back. Taking the back, loins, and buttocks as the supporting points, raise the head, hands and feet one after another. When the head lies flat, stretch the arms along the head and inhale, meanwhile raising the feet to the highest point. Exhale when raising the head and the arms and putting the legs down. While doing this, take advantage of inertia, rise up and lie down as if a seesaw. Practise it slowly at first, then quickly, and adjust the respiration method to fit the motions (use the nasal respiration method). Practise 4 to 6 times a day, 5 to 10 minutes each time.

4) Standing Straight Like a Stake Cultivation Exercise

5) Quiescent Sitting Health Cultivation Exercise

The above two exercises can be used when the general condition is getting better and after one month of practising the Relaxed and Quiescent Recumbent Exercise.

6) Expectant Point Massage

Press the Zhongwan, Tianshu, and Zusanli points each for one minute.

3. Sample Case

Ms. Zhang, 46 years old, had suffered from pain, distension in the upper abdomen, belching and a sense of prolapse for several years. She looked pale, leptosomatic and weak. Superficial gastritis accompanied with gastroptosia was diagnosed through X-ray barium meal examination. After Qigong treatment for three months, the symptoms were gradually relieved and her appetite and weight increased. Reexamination by X-ray showed that the symptoms of gastroptosia had disappeared.

VOLVULUS OF STOMACH

Volvulus of stomach often occurs when doing physical labor or playing sports. It is often found in young and middle-aged adults.

1. Clinical Manifestations

The main symptoms are pain in the abdomen, vomiting, melena, etc.

2. Qigong Treatment

1) Heaven and Earth Exercise

See the previous section of gastroptosis for details.

2) Qiaoqiao (Seesaw) Exercise

See the previous section of gastroptosis for details.

3) Massage

a. Lie on the back. Rub the abdomen with the left palm from the left to the right and then from the right to the left, 10 times respectively. Then change the right hand to do the same for another 10 times respectively. Rub slowly at first then quickly, and then slowly again. Repeat for 10 minutes.

b. Press the abdomen with the middle and index fingers from upper to lower, then from lower to upper alternately for about 2 to 5 minutes.

c. Massage the abdomen with the palms up and down and from the right to the left.

While pressing, rubbing, and massaging, make the chest, the abdomen and the buttocks rock or shake up and down to accelerate the recovery of the internal organs.

4) Others

In addition to the exercises mentioned above, jumping stairs up and down, jumping over ditches, swimming, etc, can also enhance the curative effect.

3. Sample Case

Mr. Zhou, 36 years old, had abdominal pain caused by jumping from a boat to the ground, followed by vomiting two times and melena. He had stomach trouble before. It was found in examination that there were tension and water and air noise in the upper abdomen and, upon pressing, the pain was obvious. X-ray examination showed that the location of the stomach was higher than normal, the shape was slanting, the outline was smooth, and the greater end of the stomach had turned upward, while the bulb part was upside down. The patient had severe pain after eating or strenuous movement and the implicit blood test of the excrement showed positive reaction. The X-ray reexamination one week later still showed the shape of the stomach upside down, and he was diagnosed as having volvulus of the stomach. While taking some medicine, he practised Qigong exercises, body exercises of sit-ups, and massage. Two days later, he felt no more pain, then by jumping up and down stairs, jumping over ditches and swimming for seven days, he recovered and could eat and sleep normally. The X-ray reexamination showed that his digestive tract had nothing abnormal. And he had had no relapse at the two-year follow-up survey.

CHRONIC HEPATITIS

Chronic hepatitis is a kind of chronic inflammation disease caused by many factors. The course of the disease usually lasts for more than half a year, and most cases are developed from the acute hepatitis virus. In addition, it is related to many other factors, such as chronic intestine inflammations and long-term drinking of alcoholic beverages.

1. Clinical Manifestations

Chronic hepatitis can be divided into chronic delaying hepatitis and chronic motative hepatitis. The symptoms of the former include a poor appetite, tiredness, weakness of the lower limbs, enlargement of the liver, which is painful upon being pressed. The symptoms of the latter include a pain in the liver area, dizziness, sleeplessness, long-term fever, loss of weight, abdominal swelling and pain of the joints. Both types are found abnormal in the liver functioning test at different levels.

2. Qigong Treatment

1) Relaxed and Quiescent Recumbent Exercise

2) Quiescent Sitting Health Cultivation Exercise

Practise the above exercises with the second respiration method, for 2 to 4 times a day, 30 to 40 minutes each time.

Generally, practise the Relaxed and Quiescent Recumbent Exercise first. When you begin to recover and feel stronger, you can practise the Quiescent Sitting Health Cultivation Exercise little by little and more and more.

3) Longevity Exercise

Choose the 17th, 20th and 23rd postures to practise. See Chapter Two for details.

4) Standing Straight Like a Stake Cultivation Exercise

See Chapter Two for details.

5) Six-word Respiration Exercise

Sit with glaring eyes and raising the eyebrows. Turn the head to the left and right. When the head turns to the two sides, exhale. Inhale when facing the front. Repeat for about 50 times.

6) Internal Organs Regulating Exercise

Lie on the back. Put the hands beside the navel and close the eyes. If you inhale with the nose and exhale with the mouth, make the exhaling longer. While exhaling contract the lower abdomen. If you breathe through the nose only, make the inhaling longer and float the lower abdomen. Practise 3 to 4 times a day, 15 to 30 minutes each time, no less than an hour altogether each day.

7) Three 8-Shape *Qi* Driving Cultivation Exercise

See the previous sections on chronic bronchitis and pulmonary emphysema.

8) Expectant Point Massage

Press the Zhongwan, Shuifen, and Zusanli points each for one minute.

Patients who are very weak should practise the quiescent exercise first, then the motional ones, practising the lying, sitting and standing exercises step by step according to the health condition. Later practise the quiescent and motional combined exercises, such as the Longevity Exercise to improve the endurance. In addition, the patient should keep a proper diet and avoid greasy food.

3. Sample Case

Mr. Liao, 35 years old, had suffered from pain and discomfort in the upper part of his right side accompanied with dullness, tiredness, sleeplessness, a lot of dreams, forgetfulness, yellow urine, thirst and bitter taste for 5 years. His liver function test showed abormalities and was diagnosed as having chronic hepatitis. He was hospitalized several times but did not recover. Then he began to practise Qigong. Twenty days later, he felt better and had a better appetite, slept longer, and had more strength. Three months later, all his liver function tests were normal except HBsAg. After 6 months his HBsAg test was normal, too, and all the symptoms had disappeared. His weight increased from 55 kg to 63 kg. No relapse was found in the one year follow-up survey.

CIRRHOSIS

Cirrhosis is a chronic and systemic disease characterized by damage to the liver caused by pathogenic factors which damage the liver tissues, and make the liver harden and change shape.

1. Clinical Manifestations

The patient has a poor appetite at the early stage, feels persistent and dull pain in the upper abdomen, and experiences vomiting, diarrhea, anemia, loss of weight, enlargement of the spleen, hyperfunction of the spleen and portal hypertension. At the late stage, the patient may experience ascites or massive hemorrhaging. Jaundice and spider nevus may also be found.

2. Qigong Treatment
1) Quiescent Sitting Health Cultivation Exercise
2) Relaxed and Quiescent Recumbent Exercise

Practise the above exercises 2 to 4 times a day, 30 to 60 minutes each time. The weak patient should practise for less time and step by step to avoid tiredness.

Generally, the patient who does not have serious abdominal distension and who has no ascites can practise both the above exercises alternately and breathe with the second respiration method first, then gradually change to the abdominal respiration method. Concentrate the mind on the liver or Dantian.

3) Mingmen Respiration Exercise

Stand with the feet a shoulder width apart. Lean forward, put the two hands in front of the abdomen, not touching the legs. Straight the back and pull in the chest slightly. Close the eyes for 3 minutes, and relax the front part of the body, from the head to the five sense organs, the shoulders, hands, chest, legs, and at last the feet. Repeat 3 to 4 times. Then relax the back part of body from the head to the shoulders, hands, back, waist, legs, and the feet. Repeat 3 to 4 times. Meanwhile change from the natural respiration method to the abdominal respiration method and then to the Mingmen respiration method. Keep the mind on Dantian (Qihai) point and refine the *qi* into a ball in the abdomen. Keep the mind from being too nervous. Practise 3 times a day, 30 minutes each time.

4) Three 8-Shape *Qi* Driving Cultivation Exercise

See the previous section of chronic bronchitis and pulmonary emphysema.

5) Health Cultivation Massage

See Chapter Two. Practise tapping the teeth, swallowing, and rubbing the foot arch, in order to increase the appetite and eliminate the abdominal distension.

6) Morning Walking Exercise

See Chapter Two. Practise this when you feel better and stronger to enforce the constitution

7) The Five Animals Frolic

See Chapter Two for details.

Qigong exercises have some effect on cirrhosis. Practise Relaxed and Quiescent Recumbent Exercise in bed at the beginning. When feeling better, Practise the endurance-increasing exercises to develop the constitution, such as the Morning Walking Exercise, etc. Do not practise the motional exercises when you are still weak and seriously ill.

3. Sample Case

Mr. Zhu, 48 years old, was hospitalized after a 6-hour coma. He had a history of snail fever and a 3-year history of cirrhosis. Examination and tests showed coma, ascites, abdominal varix, TTT 10 units, ZnTT 16 units, SGPT 80 units, A/G ratio reversed, external antigen of encephlitis B (-), AFP (-), and cirrhosis was found through the radio-isotope scanning. He was diagnosed as having hepatic coma, cirrhosis and ascites. After having emergency treatment for 6 months, he gradually became conscious and his liver function was improved. He was discharged from the hospital. While staying at home, he began to practise Qigong, such as the Three 8-shape Qi Driving Cultivation Exercise, and, accompanied with food treatment, he stopped smoking and drinking alcoholic beverages. One year later, his ascites disappeared, and without medicine he would not feel tired after 15 *li*'s walking.

CHOLELITHIASIS

Cholelithiasis is a kind of gallstone disease caused by cholestasis, parasitic infection of biliary tract and imbalance in metabolism of cholesterol. There are many women patients than man patients. The middle aged women, especially fat and with more children women, are easily to have this disease.

1. Clinical Manifestations

Usually, there are no obvious symptoms except a fullness in the upper and right upper abdomen, belching, vomiting of acid, abdominal distension and other symptoms of indigestion. The symptoms are more serious after meals and after having fatty food. Sometimes the patient may have gall colic, jaundice, fever, or even damage of the liver function.

2. Qigong Treatment

Qigong treatment has an effect on infrequent-attacking and less serious cholelithiasis, such as small or sand-like stones in intrahepatic bile duct and gallstone and choletithiasis without serious blocking and infection and small surviving calculus left after operations. It does not fit all cholelithiasis patients. So the patient should be careful to choose the Qigong exercises according to his own disease and constitution. In addition, the patient should coordinate the Qigong exercises with other medical treatment and diet.

1) Oxygen-inhaling Exercise

Take a deep breath in a place with fresh air. After exhaling the air completely, inhale the fresh air as much as possible. Take 10 to 20 deep breaths. It is better to jog about 1000 to 2000 metres before practising.

2) Boat-poling Exercise

The action of this exercise is just like poling a boat. As if the exerciser is standing on a boat, holding a pole in the hands and pushing the pole to the lower back direction with force to make the boat move forward. Practise 1 or 2 times a day, 30 minutes each time till you sweat. The exercise can make the thorax muscles move with force, the abdominal muscles contract and increase the moving range of the diaphragmatic muscles so as to massage the liver and gallbladder.

3) Heaven and Earth Exercise

Practise 2 to 3 times a day. See the previous section on gastroptosis for details.

4) Sail-pulling Exercise

Stand with the feet a shoulder width apart. Raise the hands above the head, with the right hand a little higher as if holding a sail rope, lift the heels and inhale at the same time. Move the hands up and down alternately as if pulling the sail down. Having pulled the sail to the level of the navel, squat down, lower the heels and at the same time exhale, contracting the abdominal and anal sphincter. After exhaling all the air, stand up. Repeat the above movement 10 to 20 times, and practise this exercise 2 to 3 times a day.

5) Crane-flying Exercise

Stand with the feet apart with the width a little more than the shoulders. Stretch the arms to each side, then bend forward to make the right hand touch the left toes, keeping the left hand up (Fig. 77). Then make the left hand touch the right toes and stretch the right hand upward. The action is like a flying crane. Cooperate the breath with the exercise rate. Repeat the movement 10 times. Practise the exercise 2 to 3 times a day.

6) Chest-striking Exercise

Stand with the feet a shoulder width apart and bend the knees slightly. Relax the whole body and breathe naturally. Clench the hands slightly. Turn the upper

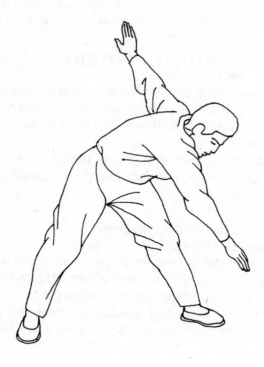

Fig. 77

body to the left and then to the right alternately with the waist as the axis. Use the inertia of the upper body's movement to strike the back and the chest with the hands alternately. The arms should be relaxed. Practise the exercise before meals till you sweat and feel relaxed and pleased.

7) Three 8-shape *Qi* Driving Cultivation Exercise

The exercise can be done together with the exercise mentioned above. Practise 1 or 2 times a day, 30 minutes each time. See the previous sections on chronic bronchitis and pulmonary emphysema for details.

8) Do some other exercises, such as walking, jogging, boating, swimming, sunbathing.

3. Sample Case

Ms. Liu, 38 years old, had suffered from abdominal pain for 4 years, getting no relief from Western medicine. She was hospitalized twice. The iodized oil roentgenograph of the gallbladder showed the image of stones of various sizes, as big as a fist altogether. Because she was afraid of operation, she turned to Qigong treatment. She practised the Longevity, Heaven and Earth, Sail-pulling and Crane-flying exercises every morning, keeping a proper diet at the same time. The symptoms disappeared after six months, and she had recovered completely one year later, with no stone images being found in the X-ray examination. She has persisted in practising the exercises for eight years and has not had a relapse since.

INTESTINAL ADHESION

Intestinal adhesion is a disease in which the intestinal surface adheres to the peritoneum in the incision after an operation and causes disturbance in the intestinal activity. It often occurs after abdominal operation.

1. Clinical Manifestations

Paroxysmal or continuous stomach aches, abdominal distension, poor appetite, dry stool, dry mouth, but don't want to drink, and poor digestive functions are the main symptoms of the disease.

2. Qigong Treatment

1) Relaxed and Quiescent Recumbent Exercise

2) Quiescent Sitting Health Cultivation Exercise

Generally, do the Relaxed and Quiescent Recumbent Exercise first and use the second respiration method. Practise 2 to 4 times a day, 30 to 60 minutes each time. When state of health and the constitution are getting better, do the Quiescent Sitting Health Cultivation Exercise and gradually come to practise both the exercises alternately. Or choose the first one to practise only till you recover. See Chapter Two for details.

3) Taiji Exercise

According to the state of health, practise Taiji Exercise in order to increase the activity and improve the constitution. See Chapter Two for details.

4. Expectant Point Massage

Press the Zhongwan, Tianshu, Zusanli, Qihai and Futong points, each for one minute, once every morning and evening.

3. Sample Case

Mr. Lu, suffered from intestinal adhesion after an operation when he was 26 years old. He felt continuous dull pain in the incision, which was 5 cm wide and 20 cm long. He had poor appetite and only ate 5 ounces food a day and experienced dizziness, acratia, sleeplessness and dry stool. Placentotherapy had no effect. Then he turned to Qigong treatment, mainly practising the Quiescent Sitting Health Cultivation Exercise and Relaxed and Quiescent Recumbent Exercise. The symptoms were relieved one month later, and disappeared completely in 100 days. He recovered fully. Since then he has been practising Qigong exercises for more than 20 years and is very healthy now.

DIARRHEA

Diarrhea is a common digestive disease. The main symptoms are increased frequency of defecation and loose stool or bloody purulent stool. When the frequency of defecation increases but the shape of the stool is normal, this is not diarrhea.

1. Clinical Manifestations

The frequency of defecation increases, the stool is loose, watery or even bloody purulent, and it is often accompanied with abdominal pain, poor digestion and other symptonms of indigestion.

2. Qigong Treatment

1) Quiescent Sitting Health Cultivation Exercise

Take the second respiration method. Practise 3 to 5 times a day and 30 to 60 minutes each time. See Chapter Two for details.

2) Expectant Point Massage

Lie on the back. Rub the palms till you feel warm, then put them on the lower abdomen and massage circularly 40 to 50 times. Then press Zhongwan, Zusanli, Yinlingquan, Guanyuan and Tianshu points each for 3 to 5 minutes. Practise once every morning and evening.

3) Taiji Exercise

Practice twice a day, 30 to 60 minutes each time. See Chapter Two.

3. Sample Case

Mr. Xiang had suffered from diarrhea since 1961. He had taken antibiotics for a long time and developed a side effect. Then he began to use traditional Chinese medicine, but it had no effect on his disease. He turned to Qigong treatment in

May 1984. The symptoms were relieved greatly three months later, and six months later he was perfectly recovered.

CONSTIPATION

Constipation is a kind of disease with dyschesia, hard stool, prolongation of the interval of defecation (usually more then 48 hours) and impediment of defecation.

1. Clinical Manifestation

The main symptoms of the disease are dyschesia, hard stool, prolongation of defecation interval, impeded defecation accompanied with abdominal distension or abdominal pain when pressed.

2. Qigong Treatment

1) Quiescent Sitting Health Cultivation Exercise

Use the second respiration method and concentrate the mind on the lower abdomen. Practise 3 to 4 times a day, 30 minutes each time. See Chapter Two for details.

2) Quiescent Recumbent Respiration Exercise

Lie on the back. Put a pillow under the head to make it as high as the chest. Close the eyes lightly, lick the palate and put the feet side by side. Press the chest with one hand and press the abdomen with the other, then take a deep abdominal breath. Inhale through the nose and make it long and deep till the abdomen goes up to push the pressing hand, then exhale slowly with the mouth. Practise 1 or 2 times a day, 50 to 100 times of breath each time.

3) Quiescent Self-massage

Lie on the back without using a pillow. Lick the palate, concentrate the mind on Dantian, and bend the legs slightly. Massage the navel region slowly and counter clockwise with the hand 50 to 100 times. Practise once morning and evening.

4) Expectant Point Massage

Massage the lower navel region with the palms circularly for 40 to 50 times, then press Zhigou, Tianshu, Zusanli and Zhaohai points each for one minute. Practise once morning and evening.

Constipation is not difficult to cure, but the ordinary treatments, such as stimulation and demulcent only have a temperary effect. If Qigong treatment is used a satisfactory effect can be achieved.

3. Sample Case

Mr. Wang, 74 years old, had suffered from poor digestion, hard stool and dysdefecation for more than 10 years. The symptoms became worse and he had constipation and diarrhea alternately and frequently. Sometimes the interval of the defecation was more than a week and a demulcent had to be used. But usually diarrhea occurred after taking it, then constipation again. No lesion was found during the surgical examination. The effect of the expectant treatment was not satisfactory and the constipation became worse. Later he turned to Qigong treatment and kept on a diet of food with more water, more fruits and vegetables and other fibre-containing food, and took some demulcent when necessary. The symptoms disappeared finally. Now his defecation is regular and he has no more diarrhea.

PROCTOPTOSIS

Proctoptosis is a kind of disease with the herniation of the anal canal, rectal mucosa, rectum and a part of the sigmoid from the anus. It is often found in children and old people.

1. Qigong Treatment

1) Anus-contracting and Qi-driving Exercise

Choose a quiet place in the early morning. Facing the east, stand with the feet a shoulder width apart and put the left hand on Dantian with the right hand above it. Close the eyes slightly and try to look at the nose tip. Touch the upper palate with the tongue. Concentrate the mind on Dantian and keep the posture for a while. Then inhale deeply and move the mind from Baihui to Chengjiang and along Renmai down to Dantian. At the same time massage Guanyuan clockwise for 2 to 5 circles to move the *qi* down to Huiyin. Then push the two hands down to the pubic symphysis. While exhaling, lift the heels and contract the muscle of buttock as much as possible and lift up the private parts. This can also lead the anus to contract and lift naturally. At the same time, concentrate the mind on *qi* and drive it to Huiyin then let it pass along anus and Chengqiang point and along Dumai to come out from Baihui on the head. Repeat it 15 times. If you can do the exercise once more in evening, the effect will be better.

Note: Beginners should be cautious about practising the exercise in the evening because it is easy to cause sleeplessness.

2) Lifting *Qi* Exercise

Lie on the back. Stretch the arms along the head, and put two or three pillows under the legs. Concentrate the mind on the Huiyin point. Use the natural abdominal respiration method. While breathing "lift" and release the reproductive organs and the anus alternately as if holding the stool and urine. The strength should be used inside not superficially. Repeat the movements 15 to 20 times each, 3 to 5 times a day.

Most patients with prolapse of the anus are weak. If they suffer only from this disease, they can have a curing effect through practising the two kinds of Qigong mentioned above and can improve their general state of health. But if the patient also has other diseases, it is necessary for him to choose other Qigong as well according to his state of health.

2. Sample Case

Mr. Cheng, 25 years old, suffered from prolapse of the anus caused by dry stool and hemorrhaging in November 1979. Later his case became serious, and even squatting would cause a prolapse from which he could recover only after rubbing and pressing slowly and gently. After being treated with the pricking pile method the hemorrhage was cured, but he still suffered from the prolapse. He started to practise anus-contracting and *qi*-driving exercises. His symptoms were gradually relieved one month later and he recovered completely three months later.

HEMORRHOIDS

Hemorrhoids is caused by the expanding of the vein's tussocks and cirsoid under the membrane of the rectal mucous and the hypodermic part of the anal canal. We can divide hemorrhoids into three types according to the area in which it occurs: internal hemorrhoids, external hemorrhoids and the mixed type. It is more common in adults.

1. Clinical Manifestations

The main symptoms are hemorrhaging, prolapse, swelling, itching, pain, a dropping feeling and the feeling of a foreign substance.

2. Qigong Treatment

1) Lifting *Qi* Exercise

Practise this 3 to 5 times a day. See the previous section of prolapse.

2) Qiaoqiao (Seesaw) Qigong

Practise this 3 to 5 times a day, 5 to 10 minutes each time. See the previous section of gestroptosia.

3) Hemorrhoid-curing Method

Standing posture a. Cross the legs, contract the buttocks, make the legs close tightly and lift the anus. Stand still with the two legs crossed, but relax the muscles of the whole body. And then contract again. Repeat this about 20 to 50 times.

b. While doing the above movement, add the respiration method to it. After inhaling enough air, hit the lower abdomen with the two loose fists and exhale at the same time. Then beat the lower abdomen from light to strong. If you feel uncomfortable, make it gentler. Repeat this for 20 to 40 times. This exercise is prohibited for pregnant and menstruating women.

c. Stand with the two legs apart and clench the fists loosely. Raise the fists through the two sides of the chest to the breast and hold up the head and chest while inhaling. After inhaling enough air, bend the upper body. Then change the fists into palms, stretch the arms backward through the two axillas (Fig. 78) and exhale deeply at the same time. Repeat 6 to 8 times.

d. Stand with two legs close. Raise the two arms along the two sides of the body. Meanwhile lift the heels and inhale deeply. Then let the arms fall naturally

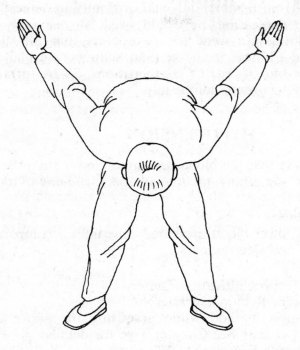

Fig. 78

in the front of the body and lower the heels exhaling deeply at the same time. Repeat 6 to 8 times.

Lying posture a. Lie on the back with the two legs crossed and relax the whole body. Contract the buttocks and thighs as tightly as possible and lift the anus with force as if holding the stool. Try to lower down the parts of the two kidneys to touch to the bed. When the exercise is done well, add the respiration method to it: Inhaling while lifting the anus and exhaling while releasing. Repeat 10 to 30 times.

b. Lie down on the bed with the two legs bent and the heels close to the buttocks. Put the two hands under the head. Taking the soles and the shoulders as the supporting point, raise the pelvis from the bed and contract the anus, inhaling at the same time. Then lower the pelvis to the bed, exhaling. Repeat 10 to 30 times.

c. Lie down on the bed, put the two arms beside the body, and relax the whole body. Raise the two arms to the upper sides and inhale at the same time till the palms of the hands reaching the highest point above the head. Then lower the arms along the front of the body to their original place. Repeat 6 to 8 times.

In a word, Qigong treatment has a satisfactory effect on less serious and early stage hemorrhoid. The patients should choose to practise it accoding to their personal state of health.

3. Sample Case

Mr. He had suffered from hemorrhoids and difficulty in defecating for more than 20 years. Whenever defecating, he would sweat all over and hemorrhage, spending 30 to 40 minutes. He went to see doctors, but all the injections, physiotherapy, traditional Chinese medicine, and acupuncture had no effect on him. He declined surgery out of fear of complications. So he turned to Qigong treatment. He has already recovered completely.

HYPOTENSION

Hypotension is a disease that the blood pressure is lower than the normal one. Its occurrence often has something to do with derangement of the vegetative nervous function.

1. Clinical Manifestations

The main symptom is lower blood pressure, sometimes accompanied by dizziness, giddiness, weakness and sleeplessness.

2. Qigong Treatment

1) Quiescent Sitting Health Cultivation Exercise

2) Relaxed and Quiescent Recumbent Exercise

Use the first respiration mathod while practising the above exercise and concentrate the mind on Dantian. See Chapter Two for details.

3) Eight Pieces of Brocade Exercise

Practise this 2 times a day, 20 to 30 minutes each time. See Chapter Two for details.

4) Sinew-transforming Exercise

Practise this 2 times a day, 20 to 30 minutes each time. See Chapter Two for details.

5) Three 8-shape *Qi* Driving Cultivation Exercise

Practise this one or two times a day, 30 minutes each time. See the previous section of emphysema.

6) Expectant Point Massage

Lie on the back and put the two arms at the two sides of the body naturally, close the eyes and relax in calm. While inhaling, recite "quiet" soundlessly and then "relax" while exhaling. Practise this 2 to 5 minutes and then begin self-massage.

a. Put the two hands on the head with the ten fingers bending and separating slightly. Massage the whole head for about 2 to 3 minutes.

b. Raise the chin up slightly. Put the palm of the left hand on the right part of the neck. Push and rub from the angle of the mandible to the neck and then to the clavicle for 8 to 10 times. Then use the right hand to do the same on the left part of the neck for another 8 to 10 times.

c. Press the arteria at the angle of the mandible with the thumb for about 5 to

6 seconds. Then rest for 10 to 15 minutes and press it again. Repeat 3 to 4 times. Then do the same on the other side.

d. Put the fingers of both hands on the forehead. Push the fingers to the two sides of the temples, rubbing them with the heels of the palms. Repeat 8 to 10 times.

e. Press Taiyang point with the two middle fingers, first gently and then forcefully, for about 5 to 6 seconds. Repeat 5 to 6 times.

f. Put the two palms on the lower chest. Inhale deeply, then press the chest while exhaling. Repeat 2 to 3 times.

7) Physical Exercise Therapy

a. Lie on the back and raise the arms. Interlace the fingers of the two hands. Inhale while pulling them away and exhale while pushing them together again. Repeat 3 to 4 times.

b. Lie on the back and put the arms at the two sides of the body. Inhale while bending the kness with the two legs together and raise the thighs as much as possible to touch the chest. Exhale while returning to the original posture. Repeat 5 to 6 times.

c. Lie on the back and inhale while bending the neck forward to make the chin touch the chest. Exhale while returning to the original posture. Repeat 5 to 6 times.

d. Sit on the bed. Turn the head to the left and then the right. Repeat 5 to 6 times.

e. Sit on the bed. Turn the upper body to the left and then right. Repeat 4 to 5 times.

f. Sit on the bed. Bend the upper body and stretch the arms as much as possible to make the hands touch the toes. Repeat 5 to 6 times.

g. Lie on the back and stretch the legs straight, keeping them close together. Raise the legs to an angle of 50 to 60 degrees while inhaling. Put them down while exhaling. Repeat 5 to 8 times.

The above Qigong exercises are helpful to reinforce the function of the cardiovascular system, to improve the process of the excitation and inhibition of the cerebral cortex and to help the blood pressure return to normal.

HYPERTENSION

Hypertension is a kind of systemic disease characterized by rising of the arterial blood pressure, accompanied by abnormal function of the heart, brain and kidney. It is also a common and frequently occurring disease and has many serious complications. It is very harmful to human health.

1. Clinical Manifestations

The occurrance and manifestations of hypertension are different in different patients. The common symptoms are headaches, dizziness, palpitation, insomnia and amnesia, and the patients are easy to be nervous, anxious, excited and tired. With the development of the disease, the heart, brain, kidney and other organs will be affected and, symptoms will occur in these organs.

2. Qigong Treatment

Qigong treatment has a good effect on high blood pressure. It can effectively induce relaxation effect and dissipate some of the mental strain factors causing high blood pressure. By relaxing, keeping one in quiescence and adjusting the cerebral cortex's function, the function of the vasomotor centre can be adjusted and the elasticity of the small arteries can be improved. In this way it is helpful in the treatment of high blood pressure. In addition, its effect of lowering blood pressure is stable and has no side effects.

1) Standing Straight Like a Stake Cultivation Exercise

Practise this 3 to 5 times a day, 30 to 60 minutes each time. See Chapter Two for details.

2) Relaxation Exercise

Take a sitting, supine lying or natural standing posture. Breathe naturally. Use the mind to relax the whole body from the top to the bottom—head, neck, shoulders, arms, hands, chest, stomach, thighs, legs, feet, soles and then concentrate the mind on Yongquan point. The idea of the exercise is to lead the qi down from the head. Repeat this for ten times. Before finishing the exercise, return the qi to Dantian and keep it there for a while. This exercise relaxes the whole body part by part. Practise 4 to 6 times a day, 20 to 30 minutes each time.

3) Six-word Respiration Exercise

Practise 1 or 2 times a day, 60 minutes each time. See the previous section of pneumatothorax for details.

4) Three 8-shape Qi Driving Cultivation Exercise

Practise 1 or 2 times a day, 30 to 60 minutes each time. See the previous section of chronic bronchitis and emphysema for details.

5) Natural Inducing Exercise

Stand naturally with the whole body relaxed and disturbing thoughts eliminated. Imagine that a gentle drizzle is falling down on your body and the rain water is flowing from the head through the body to the end of the four limbs. Imagine this 10 times.

The exercise can reduce blood pressure and relieve or get rid of the feeling of a heavy head and light feet.

Practise 3 to 5 times a day, 10 to 20 minutes each time.

6) Morning Walking Exercise

See Chapter Two for details.

7) Expectant Point Massage

First, rub the forehead with the fingers of the two hands, then rub the two sides of the head with the palms. Then press and pinch the Neiguan, Shenmen, Hegu,

Zusanli, Sanyinjiao and Xingjian points with the two hands alternately, one minute for each point. Then rub the waist with the fists and rub the stomach with the palms. At last, rub and shake the thighs and legs with the palms. Practise 2 or 3 times a day.

8) Other Qigong exercises

You can choose Longevity Exercise, Harmonization Exercise and other supplementary exercises. See Chapter Two for details.

There are many Qigong exercises which have preventive and therapeutic effects on hypertension. The patient can choose to practise according to his or her state of health and disease. Generally speaking, the quiescent exercises should be practised first, and then the motion exercises should be added as auxiliary exercises when the state of health and disease gets better.

3. Sample Case

Mr. Huang, 54 years old, had suffered from high blood pressure for more than ten years. Before he was hospitalized, his blood pressure was often above 200/120 mm Hg and he had no satisfactory effect after various treatments. He had sick leave for over a year. When he was hospitalized, his fundus examination showed oozing of blood and the electrocardiogram showed that his left ventricle was larger than normal, urine protein test +, blood NPN a little high, blood pressure 190/120 mm Hg. After two months combined treatment, mainly with Qigong, the symptoms were relieved and he was getting better. He was discharged from hospital and continued to do Qigong exercise. Three months later, his blood pressure reduced to about 160/110 mm Hg, so he tried to do some work. One year later, his blood pressure had returned normal, and remained stable at 130-140/80-90 mm Hg. Now he is able to work full time.

CEREBRAL ARTERIOSCLEROSIS

Cerebral arteriosclerosis is a kind of disease with a series of symptoms of cerebral ischemia caused by fatty substances deposited on the inner membrane of the cerebral arteries, causing pathological changes such as inner membrane hyperplasia or atheriosclerosis and resulting in the narrowness or blocking of the vessel. It is common in middle-aged and old people.

1. Clinical Manifestations

The main symptoms of the disease are dizziness, headaches, listlessness, unstable mood, distractibility, hypomnesis (very obviously), low efficiency, etc. Sometimes the patient may also have other symptoms, such as tinnitus, vomiting, changes of temper and abnormal behaviour.

2. Qigong Treatment

1) Quiescent Sitting Health Cultivation Exercise

Take the first respiration method. Practise 1 or 2 times a day, 30 minutes each time. See Chapter Two for details.

2) Longevity Exercise

Practise the 1st, 2nd, 12th, 15th, and 21st postures, 1 or 2 times a day. Refer to Chapter Two for details.

3) Sinew-transforming Exercise

Practise this 1 or 2 times a day. See Chapter Two for details.

4) Eight Pieces of Brocade Exercise

See Chapter Two for details.

5) Three 8-shape *Qi* Driving Cultivation Exercise

See the previous section of bronchitis.

The patient should choose the exercises according to his or her state of health and disease. Generally speaking, the serious patients should begin with Quiescent Sitting Health Cultivation Exercise and Three 8-shape *Qi* Driving Cultivation Exercise and then add the endurance exercises, such as Longevity Exercise and Eight Pieces of Brocade Exercise, when getting better.

3. Sample Case

Mr. Jin, 57 years old, suffered from dizziness, headaches and hypomnesis, and felt heavy in the head and light in the feet when walking. He could not walk steadily without a stick. He was diagnosed as having cerebral arteriosclerosis. After one year's treatment, there was no effect. He then turned to Qigong treatment, practising Three 8-shape *Qi* Driving Exercise once every morning and evening, and once for an hour as well as stopping smoking, tea-drinking and sex acts and eating only a vegetarian diet. Two weeks later he felt clear in the brain and did not need a stick when walking. Three weeks later, he could go up and down stairs by himself. Four weeks later, he could go out. Once after excessive exercises he suffered from insomnia. The next day he had a headache, and felt weak and dizzy and had to stay at home. Three days later, he had to be in bed because of a headache. At eight o'clock in the evening he went suddenly unconscious after experiencing a tic. But by the time the ambulance came, he had regained consciousness again. He was hospitalized for three days and diagnosed as having cerebrovascular convulsion. After being discharged from the hospital, he went to a Qigong master for treatment and practised Qigong following him. He practised Three 8-shape *Qi* Driving Cultivation Exercise no more than 30 minutes each time and Taihuzhuang (Taihu Lake Stake) Exercise no more than an hour in fresh air from 5 to 6 o'clock in the morning. Meanwhile he was on a diet of mostly vegetarian food and his weight dropped to normal in 3 months. After 6 months, he recoverd completely. Now he can jog for about 2,000 metres.

APOPLEXY SEQUELAE

Apoplexy sequelae is a kind of motion and sensory disturbance which occurs in the recovery period of a cerebrovascular accident.

1. Clinical Manifestations

After the cerebrovascular accident, the patient may experience hemiparalysis, facial palsy, sensory disturbance, lallation, etc. The above symptoms may continue after the recovery period.

2. Qigong Treatment

1) Three-line Relaxing Exercise

Take the sitting or lying posture. Breathe naturally. Relax the whole body following the mind in three lines while breathing, that is, divide the whole body into three lines, the sides, the front and the back, and relax from the top to the bottom one by one.

The first line: the two sides of the head——the two sides of the neck——shoulders——elbows——forearms——wrists——hands——fingers.

The second line: the face——neck——chest——stomach—— thighs——knees——legs——feet——toes.

The third line: the back of the head——neck——back——waist ——thighs——knees——legs——feet——soles.

Concentrate on a part, then recite "relax," then move the mind away and recite "relax" again. Start with the first line and follow the order one by one. Then do the second and the third. When you finish a line, concentrate the mind on the ending point for a while. The ending points of the three lines are the middle fingers, middle toes and the front of the soles respectively. Concentrate on these points for 1 or 2 minutes each. When you finish all the three lines, concentrate the mind on the navel for 3 to 4 minutes. Generally practise the Three-line Relaxing Exercise 2 to 3 times, then keep in quiescence for a while before finishing. Practise 3 to 5 times a day.

2) Air Bath Exercise

Take a lying or sitting posture. Relax the whole body then adjust the breath from shallow to deep and from quick to slow, and make the breaths long, deep, thin, even and stable. Adjust the breath to 8 to 10 times a minute, but do not hold the breath. Generally practise it in a room with a temperature of 25°C. Patients who can walk should practise outside. Practise 3 or 4 times a day, 5 to 15 minutes each time.

3) Self-massage

Massage yourself from the head to the face, the neck, the body and the limbs. You can do it by pushing, pinching, rubbing, etc. Massage mainly the limbs. Repeat 10 times.

4) Eight Pieces of Brocade, The Five Animals Frolic and Sinew-transforming Exercises

Choose one of the above three. Practise 1 or 2 times a day, 20 to 30 minutes each time. See Chapter Two for details.

5) Expectant Point Massage

For lower limb hemiplegia, press the part between Chengling and Baihui points on the opposite side of the head for about 30 minutes, till you feel warm in the toes of the hemiplegic leg and have sense there.

For upper limb hemiplegia, press the part between Taiyang, Heliao, Tounie and Xuanli points on the opposite side of the head till you feel warm in the fingers and have sense there. For lallation, press Shezhu point.

For difficulty in opening and closing the eyes, press the Zanzhu, Yuwei and Chengqi points.

For facial palsy, press the Qianzheng, Jiache, Xiaguan, Yifeng, Chengqi and Yangbai points.

For a twisted mouth and slobbering, press the Dicang, Chengjiang and Jiacheng points.

Qigong treatment has some effect on this disease. Patients should choose to practise according to his or her state of disease and sequelae.

3. Sample Case

Mr. Ji, 57 years old. One morning he suddenly could not speak clearly, and could not move his right hand and foot, not even get up. He was diagnosed as having apoplexy. Following the doctor's instructions, he began practising Qigong, accepting massage treatment and taking air baths and sunbaths at the same time. After a month, he could take care of himself. Then he increased the amount of exercises gradually, added therapeutic walks and practised quiescent Qigong accompanied by motion Qigong. Three months later, his blood pressure was 140/90 mm Hg and he began to do light work. After further practice for a month, he resumed his work as a fitter. Since then, thanks to persisting in such exercises as long-distance running, swimming, etc., his constitution has strengthened continually. A year later, he joined the elderly men's 5,000 metre race and won a prize.

CORONARY HEART DISEASE

Coronary heart disease (coronary arteriosclerotic heart disease) is a kind of disease caused by factors which can lead to coronary arteriosclerosis, disturb the coronary arterious blood circulation, produce a contradiction between supply and consumption, and a lack of blood and oxygen to the heart muscle. As a result, normal heart function is disturbed and the heart will change pathologically. Usually it is caused by long-term and excessive nervousness, excessive mental work and shortage of physical exercise. Coronary heart disease can be classified as latent coronary heart disease, angina, myocardial infarction and arrhythmia.

1. Clinical Manifestations

1) Latent coronary heart disease: It is common in middle-aged or old people. Usually the patient has no symptoms, such as chest distress, palpitation and

precardium stabbing pain, etc. But electro-cardiogram (ECG) examination shows ischemic change.

2) Angina: The patient feels oppressed in the lower central part of the chest, accompanied with paroxysmal strangulated pain, which may radiate to the left shoulder and arm. Sufferers can easily have an attack under the conditions of excited mood, satiation, coldness, etc. Having a rest or taking nitroglycerin tablets may quickly alleviate the pain. Attacks also take place with no apparent induction factors and display long-term pain in stillness. Nitroglycerin tablets are almost ineffective.

3) Myocardial infarction: The patient has a continuous pain or a sense of tightness in the retrosternal region or precardium. The pain may last more than half an hour, radiating to the neck, shoulders and arms. At the same time, the pain is usually accompanied by such signs as coldness of the extremities, a weak and fast pulse, low blood pressure, faint heart sound and even shock and sudden death. Most patients' ECG have specific changes.

4) Arrhythmia: This mainly includes multifocat atrial premature beat, ventricular premature beat, atrial fibrillation, parasystolic rhythm and paroxysmal tachycardia, etc.

2. Qigong Treatment

1) Relaxation Exercise and Three-line Relaxing Exercise

Adopt the lying posture, and do Relaxing Exercise or Three-line Relaxation Exercise. Breathe naturally. Practise 3 to 5 times a day, 30 to 60 minutes each time. See the previous sections of hypertension disease and apoplexy.

2) Six-word Respiration Exercise

Practise 1 or 2 times a day, 60 minutes each time. For details, see the previous section of pneumothorax.

3) Three 8-shape *Qi* Driving Cultivation Exercises

Practise 1 or 2 times a day, 30 to 60 minutes each time. For details see the previous sections of chronic bronchitis and emphysema.

4) Longevity Exercise and Morning Walking Exercise

The patient can practise these as auxiliary means of relaxation Qigong. Practise them 1 or 2 times a day, 30 to 40 minutes each time. Refer to Chapter Two for details.

5) Expectant Point Massage

Take the sitting or supine lying posture. Massage the forehead and the two sides of the head with the fingers, rub the auricles and mastoidea behind the opening of the outer ear tunnel, making those parts warm. Then press and pinch with the hands alternately the Neiguan, Shenmen, Shanzhong, Zusanli, Sanyinjiao and Yongquan points to make them gain *qi*. Finally, stand firmly, relax the arms, pound the back and the chest while turning left and right for 50 to 100 times. Repeat the above actions several times and three times a day.

In a word, the patient with the disease can achieve ideal results through practising Qigong. When choosing the specific Qigong exercises, he or she should mainly choose the quiescent ones, and the motion exercises should be used only as auxiliary ones. Because under the state of quiescence and relaxation, the total consumption and heart load decrease, the ischemia and hypoxia of the heart can improve relatively. However, adequate motion exercises can improve blood circulation, strengthen the heart and lung functions and stimulate the coronary artery to establish collateral circulation.

In addition, for those patients with arrhythmia and acute myocardial infarction, it is necessary to take medicines and go to doctor for treatment according to the state of disease.

3. Sample Case

Mr. Zhao, 53 years old. On the night of April 13, 1982, he suddenly suffered dizziness, palpitation and precardium pain, and went to hospital for emergency treatment. The examination showed that his blood pressure was 180/112 mm Hg, heart rhythm was irregular, heart beat rate was 64 to 70 times a minute, premature beat was 10 to 15 times a minute, blood cholesterol 240 mg per volume, triglyceride 196 mg per volume. ECG examination showed ischemic changes of the heart muscle and frequent atrial premature beating. He was diagnosed as having hypertension, coronary heart disease and atrial premature beating. After taking Western medicine, the premature beating still could not be eliminated completely (6 to 8 times a minute) and precardium pain occured occasionally (4 to 7 times per week). In June, he turned to comprehensive treatment with Qigong. At the beginning, he learned to practise Qigong (Quiescent Sitting Health Cultivation Qigong, etc.), accompanied by massage. After three months, his blood pressure dropped (150/90 mm Hg), precardium pain was relieved (1 to 3 times per week), and premature beat reduced (1 to 3 times a minute). And he felt well. Six months later his condition improved further and the precardium pain did not occur anymore. He resumed full-time work. He has persisted in practising Qigong for the past three years, and his condition is stable now.

CHRONIC RHEUMATIC HEART DISEASE

Chronic rheumatic heart disease is also called chronic rheumatic valvular heart disease. The main pathological change in this heart disease is chronic valve damage caused by rheumatism.

1. Clinical Manifestations

Symptoms vary according to the conditions of the valvular damage. For patients with no complications, the clinical symptoms are not obvious. The common complications are congestive heart failure and atrial fibrillation.

2. Qigong Treatment

1) Quiescent Sitting Health Cultivation Exercises

2) Relaxed and Quiescent Recumbent Exercise

When doing the above two exercises use the second respiration method and concentrate your mind on Dantian. Practise them 3 or 4 times a day, 30 to 60 minutes each time. See Chapter Two for details.

3) Relaxation Exercise

Take the lying posture. Do the Relaxation Exercise or Three-line Relaxing Exercise. Breathe naturally. Practise 2 to 4 times a day, 30 to 60 minutes each time. See the previous sections of hypertension and apoplexy sequelae.

4) Heart-recovery Exercise

Relieve yourself and rest for 15 minutes before doing the exercise. Induce the mind to be quiet gradually. Sit on a bench with the legs a shoulder width apart and put the hands on the thighs. Close the eyes slightly and make the upper part of the tongue touch the upper gum and the lower part touch the lower gum. Move the qi with the mind from the head gradually down to the feet, lowering and relaxing the arms following the qi. When the qi reaches the Yongquan points on the soles, close the eyes, at first with a small opening and then close them slightly. Concentrate the mind on the central point between the two eyes. Then move the mind down to navel. When it reaches the navel, contract the abdomen slowly and try to make both the mind and the navel touch the back of the waist. Then relax the abdomen slowly and drive the qi out of the navel. Then mentally move the qi around the navel clockwise for 36 times, first in small circles, then in large circles, and then do the same counterclockwise 24 times. Finally concentrate both the mind and the qi on the centre of the navel, and return them back to the abdomen. After holding them there for a while, relax the navel and conclude the exercise.

Practise 10 to 60 minutes each time, gradually prolonging the time of practice. After practising this kind of Qigong, you should take a walk for 20 minutes. In the period of practise, there should be no sexual activity.

5) Swallowing Qi Driving Exercise

Sit straight with the legs crossed. Put your hands on the knees. Put the tongue on the palate, knock the teeth for 36 times, stir in mouth with the tongue for five to ten times. When the saliva is full under the tongue, swallow it in five times with sound.

6) The Five Animals Frolic

7) Health Cultivation Massage

Practise the above two exercises 1 or 2 times a day, 20 to 30 minutes each time. You may choose the Five Animals Frolic according to your constitution. See Chapter Two for details.

The Qigong exercise have some therapeutic effect on the disease. Patients can also seek other medical treatment while practising Qigong. When choosing Qigong exercises, they may choose both quiescent and motion exercises. Reasonable motion exercise can improve the heart function and the constitution, on the other hand, the quiescent ones serve as the basic treatment, relieving the heart load and improving the myocardial metobolism, strengthening the cardial reserve and thereby allowing the heart function to recover.

3. Sample Case

Mr. Li, age 49. Twenty-one years ago, he was diagnosed as rheumatic heart disease, mitral stenosis and mitral incompetence (stenosis was dominated). At that time, except tiredness, other symptoms were not obvious. Five years ago he was attacked by atrial fibrillation because of excessive business trips. He was hospitalized and cured through medical threatment. One year later, atrial fibrillation occurred again. After taking medicine, fibrillation ceased. He went to Zhongshan Hospital in Shanghai for an examination, and it was suggested that he should have an operation. Being busy with his work, he did not have it. He got interested in Qigong and early in 1982 he started Qigong exercises (Rising and Dropping to Adjust the Breath Exercise, and so on). At that time, he was too weak to finish the whole exercise but gradually his strength returned and he was able to practise the exercise once in the morning and once in the evening. For the past two years he has persisted doing Qigong exercise and worked all the time without medicine. When necessary, he even works on Sunday, but his heart beat rate remains normal all the time and he is full of vigour. Hospital reexamination showed that no operation is needed.

CONGESTIVE HEART FAILURE

Congestive heart failure results from serious incompetent compensation of heart caused by a variety of diseases.

1.Clinical Manifestations

Main symptoms are dyspnea in various degrees, coughing, spitting hemoptysis, cyanosis and so on, or a decrease in urine, costalgia, bad appetite, nausea, vomiting and edema of lower limbs. Heart examination shows expansion of the left side of the heart or the whole heart.

2. Qigong Treatment

1) Quiescent Sitting and Breath-adjusting Exercise

Sit with the legs a shoulder width apart and put the hands on the thighs. Bring the ankle joint, knee joint and hip joint to 90 degree angles. Relax the shoulders, elbows, pull in the chest and contract the abdomen, close the eyes slightly and bring yourself into a quiet and relaxed state. The serious patients may sit on bed with the legs crossed. Adjust the breath consciously, adopt the natural abdominal respiration method and make the breathing deep, long, thin, smooth, stable and continuous. While exhaling, use strength to contract the abdominal muscle to make the abdominal wall sink, and move the diaphragm upward to massage the organs in the thoracic cavity. Do not hold the breath after exhaling, inhale at once, make the thorax expand and the diaphragm move downward to massage the organs in the abdominal cavity. While making the abdominal wall rise, keep the movement natural and gentle, slow and relaxed and make the exhaling longer than inhaling, at a ratio of about 3:2. Breathe 10 to 15 times a minute. Practise 5 to 15 minutes each time, once every four hours.

2) Lying Breath-adjusting Exercise

Generally this can be practised after the patient has been better for 24 to 48 hours. The patient can take the supine lying posture or latericumbent lying posture to practise the breath- adjusting exercise 2 to 3 times a day, breathing 10 times in a minute.

3) Standing Breath-adjusting Exercise

This is suitable for patients who have detumescenced and can walk about. Take the same posture as that of Standing Straight Like a Stake Cultivation Exercise (See Chapter Two for details). Breathe 8 to 10 times in a minute.

4) Walking Breath-adjusting Exercise

Do not practise this until the state of disease is better. Practise once every morning and evening 5 to 15 minutes each time. Breathe 10 to 25 times in a minute. Meanwhile, the patient can take advantage of the natural environment such as the sunlight, the air and water.

The breath-adjusting exercises are concerned with breathing on the basis of mind, with breath being the motivating power. It can improve pulmonary ventilation volume and air exchange between the blood and pulmonary cells. It can also increase the range of diaphragm lifting, massage hyperaemia heart and lungs, help blood ejection and the reflux of venous blood, and have a curing effect.

5) Sanli *Qi*-driving Exercise

Sit straight like a pine tree and steadily like a bell with the legs crossed and eyes half-closed. Look forward, relax the shoulders and put the Laogong points of the hands on the Zusanli points. Then begin to drive *qi*. Breathe with the nose, making the inhaling longer than exhaling, at a ratio of 4 to 3. Hold the end of the exhale a little longer, driving the *qi* down to Qihai point. Practise for 10 to 30 minutes.

6) Longevity Exercise

Choose the 1st and 13th postures. See Chapter Two for details.

7) Three 8-shape *Qi* Driving Cultivation Exercise

See the previous section of chronic bronchitis and emphysema.

The above two exercises can be practised as supplementary to the breath adjusting exercises.

3. Sample Case

Ms. Tan, 32 years old, had suffered from shortness of breath, coughing and palpitation for 6 years. She found it difficult to walk, so had to stay in bed and could not sleep at night. She was treated with digitalis, but refused to have an operation. After examinations she was diagnosed as having rheumatic heart disease, hyperaemia heart failure, pnemonedema and cardial function Grade II. After being treated by Quiescent Sitting Breath-adjusting Exercise, 24 hours later she could lie on her back. She turned to supine lying breath-adjusting exercise, 3 times a day, 10 minutes each time. Three days later, she could get up, walk about and take care of herself. Then she turned to Standing Straight Like a Stake Exercise. Seven days later, she was able to go back to work. Since then and for a year, she has continued practising and taking advantage of the natural environment. No relapse has been found in follow-up surveys.

CHRONIC MYOCARDITIS

Chronic myocarditis is a kind of myocardium disease caused by chronic myocardium pathological changes. Most cases occur after acute myocarditis.

1. Clinical Manifestations

The main symptoms are palpitation, shortness of breath, cardiectasis and arrhythmia, etc.

2. Qigong Treatment

1) Quiescent Sitting Health Cultivation Exercise

Practise this exercise 3 to 5 times a day, 30 to 60 minutes at a time, breathing naturally. See Chapter Two for details.

2) Three 8-shape *Qi* Driving Cultivation Exercise

See the previous sections of chronic bronchitis and emphysema.

3) Longevity Exercise

Choose the 1st and 8th postures. Practise 1 or 2 times a day, 15 to 20 minutes each time. See Chapter Two for details.

4) Morning Walking Exercise

See Chapter Two for details.

5) Eight Pieces of Brocade Exercise

See Chapter Two for details.

Qigong exercise can improve clinical symptoms without side effects. The less serious patients can practise Qigong exercises for treatment. The serious patients may accept other medical treatment while practising Qigong. Exercisers should practise the quiescent exercises first, and take the motion exercises as support.

3. Sample Case

Mr. Zhang, 46 years old, had suffered from myocarditis for 3 months. This began with fever 37.6-38.6°C, for which he could not find a cause. His heart rate was 98 beats per minute. He was hospitalized after vomiting and was diagnosed as having myocarditis. After taking medicine, symptoms were relieved, but his heart beat remained 90 per minute. He turned to Qigong exercises. One month later, his heart beat was reduced to 85 per minute, and 3 months later, was reduced to 75.

He felt well and returned to work. The one year follow-up survey showed that everything was normal.

PRIMARY THROMBOCYTOPENIC PURPURA

Primary thrombocytopenic purpura is a kind of autoimmune disease. It is common in women and young men.

1. Clinical Manifestations

The main symptoms are bleeding in the four limbs, trunk and gums, petechiaes or ecchymosis on the skin, and some times with nosebleeding and menorrhagia in women.

2. Qigong Treatment

1) Quiescent Sitting Health Cultivation Exercise

Take the first respiration method and practise it 1 or 2 times a day, 30 to 60 minutes each time. See Chapter Two for details.

2) Sinew-transforming Exercise

3) Morning Walking Exercise

4) Eight Pieces of Brocade Exercise, The Five Animals Frolic and Taiji Exercise

See Chapter Two for the above exercises. Practise 1 or 2 times a day, about 30 minutes each time.

During the acute stage of the disease, the patient can practise one of the above exercises according to condition and constitution. When the symptoms are relieved, add sunbath, coldwater bath, air bath and rope skipping, mountain-climbing, bicycling etc.

3. Sample Case

Ms. Wang, 24 years old, had suffered from purpura for 3 years. She had menorrhagia and her menstruation lasted 8 to 10 days. She sometimes had ecchymosises on the legs and failed to respond to medical treatment in several hospitals. So she could work only 6 months in a year.

She was weak with a pale face. The examination showed that she had bleeding spots all over the body, especially on the lower limbs, and the beat of her pulse was 85 per minute. According to the chemical examination she was diagnosed as having primary thrombocytopenic purpura.

She accepted Qigong treatment accompanied by other exercises, such as coldwater bath, sunbath, air bath and swimming for 2 years. Her symptoms disappeared and the chemical tests showed normal. No relapse was found in the follow-up survey.

DIAPHRAGM CONVULSION

Diaphragm convulsion (hiccuping) is characterized by the interval contraction of the diaphragm. It is commonly caused by sudden inhaling of air into the respiratory tract and the vocal cords closing.

1. Clinical Manifestations

Hiccups usually occur suddenly and continuously, and may last for several hours and even days and nights. Sometimes it attacks in intervals and lasts for several months and even interferes with the patient's talking, eating, breathing and sleeping.

2. Qigong Treatment

1) Relaxation Exercise and Three-line Relaxing Exercise

The patient can take a standing, sitting or lying posture. Do the Three-line Relaxing Exercise or Relaxation Exercise. Pay attention to relaxing the chest, waist and back repeatedly. Practise 3 times a day, 20 to 30 minutes each time. After practising the exercise, massage the Zusanli point for 5 minutes. See the previous sections on hypotension and poplexy sequelae for details.

2) Standing Straight Like a Stake Cultivation Exercise

Concentrate the mind on the fingers. Close the eyes but imagine looking at the diaphragm 15 to 20 minutes, practise 3 to 5 times a day. After ending the exercise, massage the Zusanli point for 5 minutes. See Chapter Two for details.

3) Expectant Point Massage

a. Press Neiguan point with the tips of the thumbs for about 2 to 5 minutes and Zusanli point for 2 minutes.

b. Press Shanzhong point with the pad of one of the middle fingers for 2 minutes.

c. Press Zhongwan point with a thumb tip for about one minute, repeating 2 to 3 times.

d. Press the parts above the eyeballs with the pads of the thumbs till you feel tingling.

ACROMELIC ARTERIOSPASM

Acromelic arteriospasm, also called Ragnaud's disease, is a kind of angiopathy of distal arteriolar in the ends of the limbs caused by angioneurotic dysfunction. It is common in women aged 10 to 40.

1. Clinical Manifestations

The ends of the limbs become white in symmetry and cyanosis appears, mostly on the upper limbs. Usually it appears at the fingertips at first, then spreads to the whole fingers and palms accompanied by partial sense of cold, tingling and pain, lasting for several minutes before recovery.

2. Qigong Treatment

1) Relaxation Exercise

Take the supine lying or sitting posture. Practise 3 or 4 times a day, 30 to 60 minutes each time. See the previous sections of hypotension and apoplexy sequelae for details.

2) Health Cultivation Massage
3) Sinew-transforming Exercise
4) Eight Pieces of Brocade Exercise
5) Morning Walking Exercise

Practise the above exercises 1 or 2 times a day, 15 to 30 minutes each time. See Chapter Two for details.

3. Sample Case

Ms. Sheng, 44 years old, had suffered from cold, tingling and pain on the ends of the four limbs for 20 years. She had been treated with traditional Chinese medicine and acupuncture and moxibustion, but with no effect. She practised Qigong for 2 months (Quiescent Sitting Health Cultivation Exercise, Standing Straight Like a Stake Cultivation Exercise and Eight Pieces of Brocade Exercise) and took some traditional Chinese medicine as auxiliary means. She felt tingling, warmth and swelling in the fingers, sweating at the same time—the same sense as after taking vasodilator. The exercises helped build up her strength and made her mood stable.

HYSTERIA

Hysteria is a kind of functional disorder of mental and somatic parafunction caused by some mental factors. It is common in women.

1. Clinical Manifestations

Its symptoms are complex and changable and attack momentarily with emotional characteristics, such as crying, laughing, talking, singing, dancing or keeping mum. Sometimes the patients may experience momentary faintness, dementia, paralysis, dumbness, blindness, convulsion, and etc.

2. Qigong Treatment

Qigong exercises can induce the patient into quiescence so as to reinforce and improve the function of the cerebral cortex, adjust the function of the nerve centre under the cerebral cortex and promote the suggested effect.

1) Self-inducing Exercise

Take the supine lying or sitting posture. Relax the whole body and diminish the disturbance, then induce the mind according to the state of the disease. For instance, the patient who keeps quiet may imagine that a crowd of innocent children are sitting around him or her with flowers in their hands and he or she is telling a story of a little white rabbit. This can correct the symptom of keeping quiet. A paralysis patient can induce the real (original) *qi* in the body to go down along the paralytic limbs while inhaling, and up while exhaling. Repeating this can promote the circulation of the *qi* and the blood and cure the affected limbs. Other patients can induce their minds according to their own symptoms. Practise 3 times a day, 30 to 60 minutes each time.

Self-inducing exercise is suitable to those hysteria patients who are at the stable stage and with normal consciousness. They can take advantages of language, mind, sound, temperature and illusion to relax the whole body, making the breath light, long, slow and even, diminishing the disturbance and getting into quiescence. The patients can self-induce through imagination and language and improve the pathological manifestation through psychological adjustment. While practising, make sure that the mind and sound should be gentle and natural and not in a hurried or forced way.

2) Eight Pieces of Brocade Exercise

Practise 1 or 2 times a day, 20 to 30 minutes each time. See Chapter Two for details.

3) Longevity Exercise

Practise the 1st and 15th postures 1 or 2 times a day, 30 minutes each time. See Chapter Two for details.

4) Sinew-transforming Exercise

Practise 1 or 2 times a day, 30 to 45 minutes each time. See Chapter Two for details.

FACIAL NERVE PARALYSIS

Facial nerve paralysis is caused by ischemia. It often occurs after long-time stimulation of cold wind. It is common in people aged 20 to 40, and more common in men.

1. Clinical Manifestations

It usually attacks suddenly at night. The patient's eyelids and lips are found inflexible the next morning. When the patient rinses the mouth, water will spill over the corner of the mouth.

2. Qigong Treatment

1) Relaxed and Quiescent Recumbent Exercise

Relax and keep quiescent naturally. Concentrate the mind on Dantian. Make the breathing deep, long, thin, even and slow. Combine the original *qi* inside the body with the air outside, making it internal *qi* and driving it along the whole body. See Chapter Two for details.

2) Three 8-shape *Qi* Driving Cultivation Exercise

Take a sitting, lying or standing posture. Practise 3 times a day, 30 minutes each time. See the previous sections of chronic bronchitis and emphysema.

3) Knocking Exercise

Knock at the effected part of the face with the bent index finger or index and middle fingers. Knock the Taiyang, Xiaguan and Jiache points mainly, and also the Yangbai and Tinggong points. Knock quickly, evenly and rhythmically but not too fast. Make the muscle vibrate and the strength go deep and spread all around.

4) Expectant Point Massage

Press, rub and pinch the Taiyang, Dicang, Jiache, Hegu and Yingxiang points on the affected side of the face 5 to 10 minutes each time, once in the morning, once in the evening.

3. Sample Case

Mr. Yao, 61 years old, suddenly found that water spilled over his left mouth corner and he could not close his left eye when brushing the teeth one morning. Different treatments had no effect on him. He turned to Qigong. After practising Qigong exercises for one month (mainly the Three 8-shape *Qi* Driving Cultivation Exercise), the two sides of his face became symmetrical when speaking, although the left part of his face remained less flexible. Six months later, he had recovered completely.

RHEUMATOID ARTHRITIS

Rheumatoid arthritis is a kind of chronic systemic disease with poly, arthritis as its main manifestation. All the joints of the body can be eroded, especially the joints on the four limbs. In serious patients, spinal and sacroiliac joints may be eroded besides the limb joints. It is common in young and middle-aged people.

1. Clinical Manifestations

Patients have wandering and symmetric pain and swelling in the small joints on the limbs. The joints gradually become stiff and dysfunctional. In the later stage, the patient may experience muscle atrophy, stiffness in the joints and deformity of the limbs and trunk.

2. Qigong Treatment

1) The Five Animals Frolic

Practise 2 or 3 times a day, 30 minutes each time. See Chapter Two for details.

2) Eight Pieces of Brocade Exercise

Practise 1 or 2 times a day, 30 minutes each time. See Chapter Two for details.

3) Expectant Exercise

Choose the exercises for the parts of the neck, spine, shoulders, elbows, hips and knees in order to correct the deformity and improve their function.

a. Stretching the chest and arms: Take the standing posture. Hold the chest with the two arms and then stretch them to the two sides. Repeat 3 to 5 times.

b. Lifting the arms: Take the standing posture. Put the hands on the abdomen first and then lift them up in the two sides of the body till the palms touch each other, then lower the arms and put the hands back on the abdomen. Repeat several times.

c. Facing upward: Stand with one foot in front of the other. Put the hands on the back of the head, throw out the chest and face upward. Repeat several times.

d. Akimbo bending sideward: Stand with the arms akimbo. Lift one arm above the head while bending the waist sideward. Then do the same with the other arm. Repeat several times.

e. Stretching the arms backward: Stand with one foot in front of the other. Lift one arm and stretch it backward as far as possible, then lower the arm. Exchange the position of the feet, stretch the other arm. Repeat 3 to 5 times.

4) Exercise in Water

Arthritis patients can also soak the joints of the fingers, wrists, elbows and ankles in warm water and do swimming exercises. By taking advantage of the water buoyancy and the wave action, it is possible to prevent and treat various arthirits diseases. If possible, the patients can bathe in warm water or a hot spring. Warm water (at the temperature of 37°) can relieve muscle pain and contracture, make the blood vessels of the skin contract and diastole, diminish inflammation, kill pain and prevent muscle and joint deformity.

5) Palm and Finger Exercise

This is done mainly to prevent and treat wandering pain, muscle contracture and joint stiffness of the small joints of the hands.

a. Thumb turning: Hold the hands as fists, turning the thumbs from left to right 50 to 100 times.

b. Standing up and bending down: Stretch the hands with the fingers closed, then bend the wrist down, making all the fingers close together like a hook for 30 to 50 times.

c. Palm swinging: Stretch the hands and swing them from the left to the right 30 to 50 times.

d. Fitting balls: Hold two iron balls in one hand and revolve them. If you have no iron balls, two large walnuts or two table-tennis will do. Revolve them 100 to 200 times in one hand and then change to the other hand.

e. Clenching the fists to increase the strength: Clench the fists, then stretch the hands. Repeat 30 to 50 times.

f. Revolving the fists: Clench the fists, taking the wrists as the axis. Revolve them 50 to 60 times.

6) Longevity Exercise, Sinew-transforming Exercise and Morning Walking Exercise.

Practise 1 or 2 times a day, 30 minutes each time. See Chapter Two for details.

The patient should choose the Qigong exercise according to the affected parts and the state of the disease. The patient can take walking, jogging, climbing mountains and other sports as auxiliary means. In order to prevent humpback and other deformities caused by rheumatoid arthritis, the patient should sleep with a low pillow and on wooden beds.

3. Sample Case

Ms. Kong, 38 years old, had suffered from rheumatoid arthitis for 6 years. Her finger joints, wrists and ankles were swollen and ached. The hospital examination showed that her wrist joints were stiff, finger joints were swollen, anti-0 833 units, blood sedimentation 18 mm/hr, rheumatoid factors positive criteria. She was treated with acupuncture, indomethacine and other traditional Chinese medicine, but this had no effect and she could not work. She turned to Qigong exercises, mainly practising the Longevity Exercise. Three months later, the pain died away. She went on practising Qigong for another 6 months, during which there was no relapse. She went back to work and experienced no relapse in the following 2 years.

CERVICAL SPONDYLOPATHY

Cervical spondylopathy is a common disease caused by the retrogressive pathological changes of the vertebra and intervertebral discs. When it attacks, the cervical nerve root, spinal cord and the soft tissue around are pressed and stimulated, resulting in pain and numbness in the neck, shoulders and arms. It is common in middle-aged and old people.

1. Clinical Manifestations

It is a delayed type disease and less serious at the beginning. Usually the patients feel indisposition and intermittent pain on the neck and shoulders. The pain gradually spreads to one arm, after which the fingers feel cold and as if being shocked by electricity. Some serious patients may feel burning pain in the arm.

2. Qigong Treatment

1) Longevity Exercise

Practise 1 or 2 times a day, 20 minutes each time. See Chapter Two for details.

2) Turning Exercise

a. Turning the head to the left and right: Take the standing or sitting posture. Turn the head slowly to the left and then the right as much as possible. When reaching the farthest point, return a little, then go even farther. While turning, the sight should go with the head, looking backward or upper backward (Fig. 79). Turn 8 to 12 times to each side.

b. Facing upward: Take the standing or sitting posture with the arms akimbo. Move the head backward to face upward and look at the sky. Enlarge the range of the action gradually as much as possible (Fig. 80). Repeat 8 to 12 times.

c. A trial of strength between nape and arms: Take the standing or sitting posture. Put the hands on the nape with the fingers crossed to support the head. Push the head backward while pulling it forward with the hands, opposing the two for a while. Then return to the original posture (Fig. 81).

d. Turning round and looking back: Stand in the left bow step. Turn the upper part of the body to the right. At the same time, hold the left palm up, stretch the

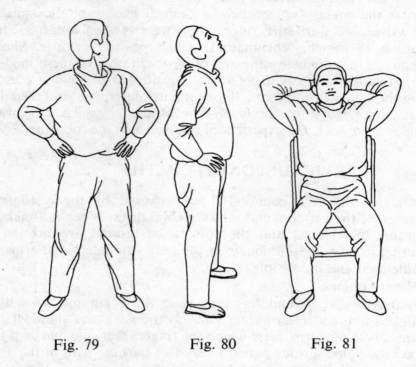

Fig. 79   Fig. 80   Fig. 81

right hand down as much as possible and turn the head to the right to look at the right hand (Fig. 82). Then return to the original posture. Stand in the right bow step to do the same oppositely. Repeat 8 to 12 times.

e. Turning the neck: Take the standing or sitting posture. Breathe naturally, relax the head and neck then slowly turn the head and neck as much as possible (Fig. 83), clockwise and counterclockwise alternately for 6 to 8 times.

f. Massaging the neck: Take the standing or sitting posture, massaging the neck with the two hands alternately 20-30 times.

The main point of the above six exercises is to practise them slowly and in a large range. After each exercise, the patient should rest for a while. Do not practise continuously. Practise 1 or 2 times a day, 10 minutes each time.

3) Longevity and Taiji exercises

Choose some of the sections or the complete set to practise, 1 or 2 times a day, 20 minutes each time. See Chapter two for details.

4) Take swimming, sun bath and airbath as auxiliary means.

5) Expectant Point Massage

Press the Jingzhong, Quchi and Yangxi points for one minute each, two times

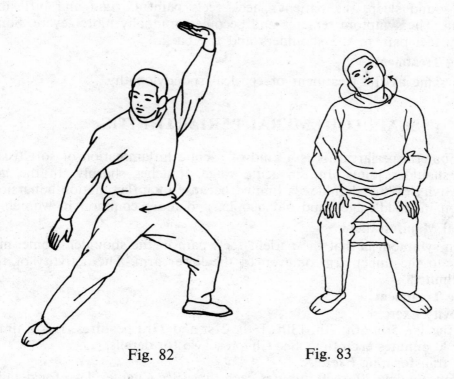

Fig. 82   Fig. 83

a day.

3. Sample Case

Mr. Yang, 48 years old, had suffered from pain on the neck and shoulders and numbness on the index and middle fingers for more than one year. X-ray examination showed hyperostosis on his fifth to seventh cervical spine. His head and neck could not turn left and he felt numbness in the left shoulder and the left upper arm and could not drop it for long. He was diagnosed as having disorder of the small joints of the cervical spine. He was treated with massage and Qigong exercises. He practised the Longevity Exercise for 15 minutes and swam for 30 minutes every morning. His symptoms were relieved before long. He now moves normally.

STIFF NECK

Stiff neck is caused by sleeping in a wrong position or sleeping outside in a windy night. Although the symptoms can improve naturally, it takes the less serious patients 3 to 5 days, and the serious patients weeks.

1. Clinical Manifestations

After a sound sleep, the patient's neck feels painful, rigid and inflexible when turning. The symptom remains and becomes gradually more severe. Some patients may feel pain in the shoulders and the back.

2. Qigong Treatment

It is the same as the treatment of cervical spondylopathy.

SCAPULOHUMERAL PERIARTHRITIS

Scapulohumeral periarthritis is a kind of aseptic inflammation of soft tissue around the shoulder joints. In the acute stage, it aches sharply. In the late stage, the activity of the shoulder is limited because of inflammation adhersion. It is common in middle-aged and old people, and more common in women.

1. Clinical Manifestations

The main symptom is that the patient feels pain in the shoulder. Sometimes pain spreads to the upper arm or even to the lower arm. The activtity of the shoulder is limited.

2. Qigong Treatment

1) Longevity Exercise

Practise the 1st, 5th, 6th, 7th, 13th, 16th, 21st and 23rd postures, 1 or 2 times a day, 20 to 30 minutes each time. See Chapter Two for details.

2) Sinew-transforming Exercise

Practise once a day, 20 to 30 minutes each time. See Chapter Two for details.

3) Taiji Qigong

See Chapter Two for details.

4) Taiji Heaven Exercise

a. Stand in relaxation and quiescence with the feet a shoulder width apart. Keep the mind in quiesence and concentrate it on all the things in heaven and earth. Keep the head straight, close the eyes slightly, lick the palate with the tongue, close the mouth slightly, drop the shoulder and elbows, pull in the chest a little, draw the abdomen, relax the hips, make the crotch a circle, bend the knees slightly.

b. Stand with horse riding posture. Clench the fists loosely and put them close to the waist with palms up. Stretch the fists forward and exhale. Turn the palms down and return them to the waist—inhaling. Repeat 10 to 15 times.

c. Stand and stretch the hands up above the head with the fingers interlaced and the palms up. Taking the waist as the axis, turn the upper part of the body from the front, to the right, the back and the left as a circle. Breathe once every circle. Exhale when bending forward and inhale when bending backward. Turn clockwise and counterclockwise, 5 to 10 times each.

d. Stand and put the hands back on the waist. Raise the right hand above the head with the palm up. At the same time, step a half step forward with the right foot. At the same time move the weight forward and raise the left heel off the ground—inhaling. Return to the original posture while exhaling. Change to the other hand and foot and do the same. Repeat 15 to 20 times.

e. Stand with the arms dropped. Turn the right arm around from the upper-front to the lower back, lifting the right foot off the ground and inhaling. When the hand close to the knee, begin exhaling. Change to the other arm and leg, doing the same. Repeat 10 to 15 times.

f. Stand with the feet a little wider than a shoulder width apart. Bend the knees and clench the fists loosely. Raise the fists to the height of the shoulders with the palms inward. Then raise the arms higher with the hands stretched and the palms forward. Raise the head to look at the fingers, lifting the heels from the ground, throwing out the chest, drawing the abdomen and inhaling at the same time. Return to the original posture. Repeat 10 to 15 times.

5) Other shoulder-joint movements and sports

Patients can practise arm turning and swinging exercises, swimming, massage and sports apparatus exercises. The moving range should gradually work from small to large. Practise several times a day.

Qigong exercises and sports have a satisfactory effect on scapulohumeral periarthritis. They can speed up recovery.

3. Sample Case

Mr. Qian, 40 years old, suffered from pain and dysfunction on the right shoulder for 3 months. He felt pain in the right shoulder when raising the right arm outward, turning it back and raising it forward and needed help when dressing and undressing. After examination, he was diagnosed as having scapulohumeral periarthritis. He accepted Qigong treatment, mainly practising the Longevity Exercise. After one week he felt better. Three weeks later, he could put on and take off his clothes himself. He went on practising Qigong exercises, with other sports as auxiliary means, for 5 to 10 months. No relapse was found in the 2-year follow-up survey.

TENNIS ELBOW

Tennis elbow, also called external humeral epicondylitis, is a common chronic strain disease caused by chronic strain of the common tendon of the extensor muscle and tissues of the forearm.

1. Clinical Manifestations

The patients feel pain on the external elbows, more severe after labour and obvious when pressed. The grip strength decreases.

2. Qigong Treatment

1) Longevity Exercise

Choose the 1st, 4th, 9th and 21st postures. Practise 1 or 2 times a day, 15 to 20 minutes each time. See Chapter Two for details.

2) Taiji Heaven Exercise

Practise 1 or 2 times a day, 15 to 20 minutes each time. See the previous section of scapulohumeral periarthritis.

3) Massage

Massage the pain points and the around tissue dozens of times. Raise up, drop down, swing forward and backward and stretch sideward the arms dozens of times, and then pinch, press, rub and tap with fingers for ten times each, coordinate the movement and the respiration method. Repeat until you feel pain on the affected part, then massage it gently.

3. Sample Case

Ms. Zhou, a 16-year old table tennis player, had suffered from tennis elbow for more than a month and could not continue training. Even washing the face, wringing a towel and carrying a basin caused sharp pain. Sometimes she was even awakened by the pain. She began practising the longevity and other Qigong exercises, accompanied with massage. After one course of treatment, the pain was relieved and she could go on training. Two courses later, she had recovered completely. Now she is continuing to practise Qigong exercises to strengthen the effect.

MYOTENOSITIS OF COMMON EXTENSOR MUSCLE OF THE FINGERS

Myotenositis of common extensor muscle of the fingers is caused by overloading or long and chronic strain of the common extensor muscle.

1. Clinical Manifestations

The main symptom is pain in the wrist and arm when moving, especially when wringing a towel or carrying a basin.

2. Qigong Treatment

Qigong treatment is usually used after the failure of other treatments, such as medicated plasters, medicine, physical treatment and cold and warm wet dressing.

1) Longevity Exercise

Choose the 1st, 4th, 11th, 16th and 21st postures. Practise two times a day, 30 minutes each time. See Chapter Two for details.

2) Palm and Finger Exercise

See the previous section of rheumatoid arthitis.

3) Penguin Exercise

Stand with the two feet a shoulder width apart. Raise the arms higher than the shoulder joints with the elbows bent, hands dropped and the palms outward (Fig. 84). Swing the shoulders up and down alternately and make the body rock, with

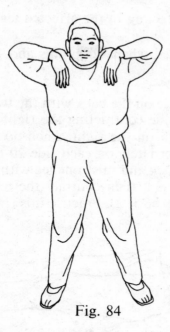

Fig. 84

the heels lifted alternately following this. Coordinate the respiration with this. Rock 30 to 50 times at a rate of 15 times a minute.

3. Sample Case

Mr. You, 48 years old, suffered from wrist pain and had not been able to wring towels for two months. There was no effect after some medical treatment. The examination showed that there was no obvious swelling on the local part, but that he felt obvious pain when pressed. When he clenched the fists, a rubbing sound could be heard clearly from the forearms. He was diagnosed as having myotenositis of the common extensor muscle of the fingers and began Qigong treatment. He practised the Longevity Exercise in the morning and evening, each time for 30 minutes, and the Palm and Finger Exercise during breaks. One week late, he no longer felt pain. Now he is continuing to practise Qigong exercises. No relapse was found at the half-year follow-up survey.

PROLAPSE OF LUMBAR INTERVERTEBRAL DISC

Prolapse of the lumbar intervertebral disc, also called prolapse of the nucleus pulposus of the lumbar intervertebral disc, is common in young and middle aged people. Patients feel pain on one side of the waist and leg. If not treated in time, it will affect the living and working of the patient.

1. Clinical Manifestations

The main symptom is pain on one side of the waist and radiating pain in one leg, or a numb, cold and swollen feeling in the affected leg.

2. Qigong Treatment

Qigong exercises should be used when symptoms and signs are relieved after massage treatment.

1) Waist-treating Exercise

a. Hip bone moving exercise: Lie on the back with the two legs straight. Stretch the left leg forward with force while contracting the right leg backward to make the pelvis low on the left and high on the right. Then do the same on the other side (Figs. 85-1, 2, 3). Practise alternately on each side 20 to 30 times.

b. Foot stamping: Lie on the back and raise one leg with the knee bent as much as possible. Kick the leg out straight, then contract the muscles of the leg for a while and then bring it down (Figs. 86-1, 2). Practise this first with the healthy leg,

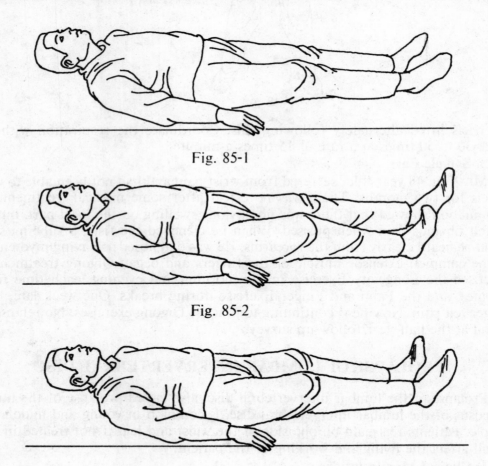

Fig. 85-1

Fig. 85-2

Fig. 85-3

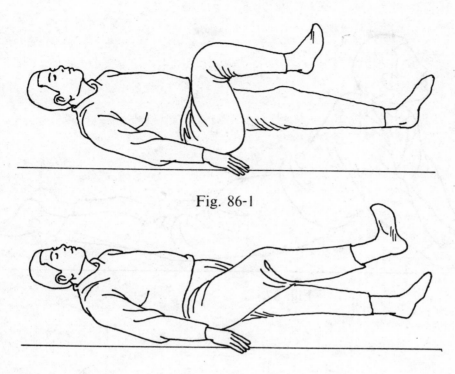

Fig. 86-1

Fig. 86-2

then with the affected leg alternately 20 to 50 times.

c. Lie prostrate with the two hands holding the bed. Raise the head and the upper body with the support of the hands, so as to make the chest stick out as much as possible. Make the strength reach the waist (Fig. 87). Lie down to rest for a while. Repeat 5 to 10 times.

d. Swallow posture: Lie prostrate. Stretch the arms and legs backward. Raise the upper body and legs simultaneously looking like a flying swallow (Fig. 88). Don't bend the knees. Hold this for about a minute. Then lie down to rest for a while. Repeat 3 to 5 times.

2) Up-and-Down Respiration-adjusting Exercise

Stand with the feet a little more than a shoulder width apart. Raise the hands with palms downward slowly along the front of the body, inhaling at the same time. When the palms reach the highest point turn them up. Inhale sufficient air and throw out the head backward. Hold this for a short time, then exhale while lowering the hands to the sides of the body, and squat down and the hands touch the ground. Exhaling all the air in the lungs, rise up slowly. Repeat for 3 to 15 minutes.

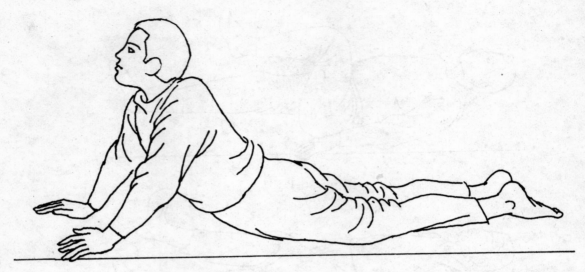

Fig. 87

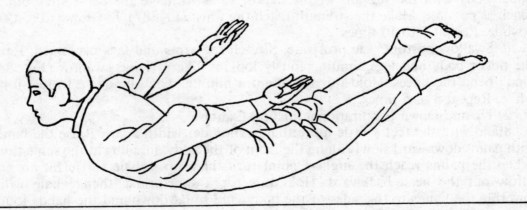

Fig. 88

3) Respiration-adjusting and Waist-strengthening Exercise

Before going to bed in the evening, sit on the bed with the legs stretched, hands on hips. Bend the waist forward and stretch the arms slowly to touch the toes. Then sit straight, concentrate the mind and the respiration on Mingmen point on the waist. Repeat 18 times. Then lick the palate and use the abdomen respiration method. While inhaling, imagine looking at Baihui point on the head. Hold the breath for a while and contract the anus. Then exhale and concentrate the mind on Mingmen and Shenyu points on the waist. Breathe like this for 36 times. Then massage Mingmen and Shenyu with the palms for 36 times and massage the lumbar vertebra with the fists for another 36 times. Repeat this till you feel warm on the waist.

4) Taiji Qigong and Longevity Exercise

Practise 1 or 2 times a day, 20 to 30 minutes each time. See Chapter Two for details.

3. Sample Case

Mr. Zhang, 61 years old, had suffered pain on the waist and disturbance of the waist activity since 1975. And the lower limbs were radiated. He was diagnosed as prolapse of the lumbar intervertebral disc, the fifth lumbar vertebra sacralization and the false joint's formation caused by the enlargement of the left spinous process and the sacrum ala. He was treated with traditional Chinese and Western medicine, but had no obvious improvement. Later the muscles on his legs became atrophied, and he felt severe pain and had to stay in bed. Then he turned to Qigong treatment—practising mainly on the bed. He took some oral traditional Chinese medicine and massage treatment as auxiliary means. Forty days later, the symptoms were obviously relieved and he could walk downstairs to practise Qigong exercises outside. Half a year later, the symptoms basically disappeared. Now he is able to play basketball, ride a bicycle and play other sports games.

ACUTE LUMBAR SPRAIN

Acute lumbar sprain is a common injury. It is common in young and middle-aged people and occurs more in physical workers or in people who seldom take part in physical labour when they do it occasionally. It is often caused by incorrect posture when moving something heavy, slipping or excessive movement, such as bending forward and backward and turning, surpassing the normal physiological limitation of the waist, resulting in the injury of the muscles, ligaments, joints, synovium and other soft tissues of the waist and buttocks.

1. Clinical Manifestations

After the injury, the patient feels pain and stiffness in one or both sides of the waist. It is difficult for the patient to bend, turn, get out of the bed and even turn the body over in bed. The patient experiences muscle spasms in the waist and feels pain when pressed. X-rays show no pathological changes.

2. Qigong Treatment

Usually an acute lumbar sprain patient should stay in bed and rest for 1 or 2 days. Qigong treatment should be adopted when severe pain has eased.

1) Up-and-down Respiration-adjusting Exercise

Practise 1 or 2 times a day, 10 minutes each time. See the previous section of prolapse of lumbar intervertebral disc.

2) Respiration-adjusting and Waist-strengthening Exercise

Practise 1 or 2 times a day, 5 to 15 minutes each time. See the previous section of the prolapse of lumbar intervertebral disc.

3) Kneeling Exercise

Kneel on the ground with the two arms stretching forward and the two hands touching the ground. Turn the waist and the lumbar vertebra to make them relaxed and gain *qi*. Stretch the waist and spine further forward, then throw the upper body backward. After repeating 18 times, you may feel the cold air being exhausted from the backbone. Then massage the waist for 36 times.

4) Waist-drawing Exercise

a. Adjusting legs: Stand on one foot with one hand holding something to support the body. Stretch the other leg and lift it as high as possible (Fig. 89). When reaching the highest point, hold it for a while and bend the body forward until you feel tingling and strain on the back of the thigh and the hip, then put the leg down. Change to the other leg to do the same. Repeat 5 to 10 times alternately.

b. Leg-pressing: Stand on one leg put the other leg on a table or something as high as your hip joint so as to bend the hip joint as about a 90 degree. Stretch the arms forward to make the hand touch the toes (Fig. 90). Hold this for a while till the popliteal fossa and the hip feel severe tingling and strain. Then put it down and change to the other leg to do the same. Repeat 5 to 10 times alternately.

c. Buttock-raising: Lie on the back. Bend the knees and raise the buttocks so as to have the feet and shoulders supporting the body (Fig. 91). Contract the muscles of the waist and back continuously, holding like this for a while. Then lower the buttocks down to rest for a while. Repeat 3 to 10 times.

LUMBAR MUSCLE STRAIN

Lumbar muscle strain, also called functional waist pain, chronic injured waist pain and kidney weakness waist pain, usually is caused by external injury, incorrect sleeping posture and some congenital defects, and is often found in adults.

1. Clinical Manifestations

The patient feels pain at one side or both sides of the waist, sometimes the pain is severe and sometimes weaker. It becomes worse after a long period of standing or sitting or overwork. After a rest, the pain will be relieved. Sometimes the patient

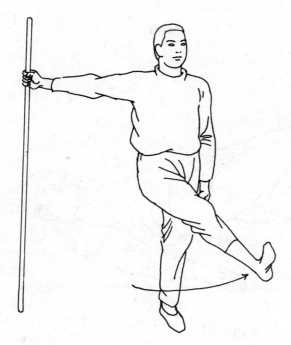

Fig. 89

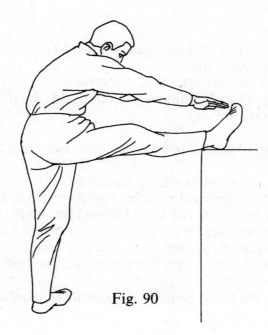

Fig. 90

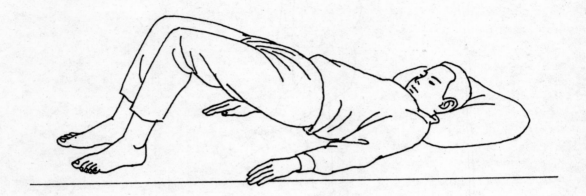

Fig. 91

may also have such symptoms as scoliosis, lumbar muscle spasms and lower limb aches.

2. Qigong Treatment

1) Waist-treating Exercise

Practise 1 or 2 times a day, 15 to 30 minutes each time. See the previous section of prolapse of lumbar intervertebral disc.

2) Breath-adjusting and Waist-strengthening Exercise

Practise 1 or 2 times a day, 15 to 30 minutes each time. See the previous section of prolapse of lumbar intervertebral disc.

3) Waist-drawing Exercise

Practise 1 or 2 times a day, 10 to 20 minutes each time. See the previous section of acute lumbar sprain.

4) Abdomen-contracting and Waist-lowering Exercise

Lie on the back. Tense the abdominal muscles and iliopsoas muscles in order to force the lumbar vetebra to touch the bed. Meanwhile, limit the abdominal respiration method and use more natural chest respiration method, but don't hold the breath. Keep this state as long as possible, according to your own constitution. Return the original posture and rest for a while when you are tired.

5) Counter-walking Exercise

a. Relax all the muscles in the body, bend the knees a little, then walk backward with the same pace as you walk forward. While walking, clench the fists with the four fingers covering the thumb, and swing the arms back and forth gently and naturally.

b. Arms akimbo with the thumbs backward and other fingers forward, press the thumbs on the Shenyu points and massage the points once every step. While walking backward, inhale through the nose and exhale through the mouth naturally, making the exhaling longer.

Practise once every morning, 5 to 6 minutes each time, walking for about 100 to 300 steps.

6) Longevity Exercise, Sinew-transforming Exercise, Eight Pieces of Brocade Exercise, the Five Animals Frolic and other Qigong exercises can be practised according to the constitution and state of illness of the patients. See Chapter Two for details.

3. Sample Case

Ms. Zhu, 55 years old, suffered from waist pain on the left side, which could be relieved only after rubbing for several times. In recent years, the pain got worse and spread to the buttocks and thighs, especially in the rainy season and changable weather. The pain was often accompanied by tingling and swollenness making her incapable of standing for a long time. After the hospital examination, she was diagnosed as having lumbar muscle strain. She began to practise Qigong exercises and often massaged the waist herself. The symptoms were relieved a month later. By three months later she had recovered, returned to work and was doing some housework as well. Now she is continuing the Qigong exercises to strengthen the curative effect.

SCIATICA

Sciatica is characterized by pain in the buttocks, back of the legs where the sciatic nerves branch. It is common, especially in middle-aged people.

1. Clinical Manifestations

Usually the patient feels dull, burned or sharp (as if being cut) pain along the area where the sciatic nerves branch, such as in the buttocks, the back of the thighs and shanks and the popliteal space. The pain becomes worse when it is cold or the patient suffers from a cough or does physical exercise.

2. Qigong Treatment

1) Standing Straight Like a Stake Cultivation Exercise

Use the natural respiration method and concentrate the mind on the affected part. If the patient feels burning pain, imagine experiencing cold, snowy weather or the cold wind in an air-raid shelter. If the patient feels dull or sharp pain as if being cut, imagine being in a warm and comfortable place. See Chapter Two for details.

2) Sinew-transforming Exercise and the Five Animals Frolic.

Practise twice a day and 30 minutes each time. See Chapter Two for details.

3) Breath-adjusting and Waist-strengthening Exercise

Practise 1 to 2 times a day, 15 to 30 minutes each time. See the previous section of prolapse of lumbar intervertebral disc.

4) Pushing and Drawing Exercise

Stand with one foot in front of the other and put hands to one side of the body positioned as if holding a ball. Lean the body backward with the back foot as the supporting point, and inhale at the same time (Fig. 92). Then bend the body forward a little, pushing the imaginary ball to the front and exhale. Repeat 16 times. Then put the hands in the other side of the body to do the same. Exchange the hands 2 to 4 times.

5) Net-drawing Exercise

Stand with one foot in front of the other and imitate the action of drawing a fishing net with two hands. At the beginning bend the body forward a little with the heel of the back foot off the ground and inhale while drawing the net up. Lower the heel and straight the body. Then exhale while drawing the net back, leaning

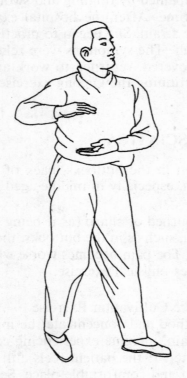

Fig. 92

the body backward with the heel of the front foot off the ground. Repeat 10 times, then change to the other side to do the same.

6) Expectant Point Massage

a. Rub the surface of Qihai point 100 times, then press it a little and rub it another 100 times. Then press with force and rub still another 100 times. Use the building-up massage method in the above rubbing (See Chapter Five for the building-up and letting- out massage method). Press three times with three breaths (see the following section of lung cancer for the method of pressing three times with breaths, but pay attention to exhaling before inhaling). Then put the hand on the affected part and use the letting-out massage method to rub 100 times with force, another 100 times with less pressure and still another 100 times on the surface of the skin. Press 3 times with 3 breaths.

b. Press the Zusanli and Yinlingquan points for one minute to make them gain *qi*.

In a word, the sciatica patient should practise Qigong with the combination of quiescent and motional exercises. Female sciatica patients should not practise this exercise when they are pregnant.

3. Sample Case

Mr. Dong had suffered from sciatica for three years. He felt pain from the left ankle to the buttocks, which was more severe when it was overcast or rainy. It was hard for him to walk, stand and sit, and he could not carry heavy things. He was treated in several hospitals without effect. He turned to Qigong exercise, mainly practising The Five Animals Frolic. In the first two months he had without effect, but in the third and fourth months, his symptoms were relieved. Half a year later, he had recovered completely and returned to work.

OSTEOPHYTE

Osteophyte is a common disease which can often be found in old people. Sometimes it may last for a long time and is hard to cure. The patients suffer unbearable pain which affects their work and lives.

1. Clinical Manifestations

The main symptoms are that the patients may feel numbness, dullness and pain. Sometimes the symptoms are relieved after sports exercises.

2. Qigong Treatment

At the beginning of practising Qigong exercise, the patient may take some medicine as an auxiliary means. After 1 or 2 months later, the patient can reduce the amount of the medicine gradually to increase Qigong exercise.

1) Quiescent Sitting Health Cultivation Exercise

Practise 2 or 3 times a day, 30 to 60 minutes each time. See Chapter Two for details.

2) Longevity Exercise

Practise once a day, 30 to 60 minutes each time. Choose the postures to practise according to the positions of osteophyte, such as the 2nd, 9th and 19th postures. See Chapter Two for details.

3) Three Cores Together Exercise

Conbine the mind with the *qi* and sit in relaxation and quiescence with the hips, knees and ankles bent at an angle of 90 degrees. Rub the hands till they are warm, put one ankle on the knee of the other leg, put one hand on the knee and press the palm of the other hand on the sole of the foot, and meanwhile concentrate the mind on Huxin (centre of the lake). Then rub the sole of the foot 50 to 100 times, clockwise and counterclockwise respectively. Breathe with each rub. Then change to the other hand and foot to do the same.

4) Sinew-transforming Exercise and The Five Animals Frolic

Practise these as auxiliary exercises, choosing according to the patient's constitution. Don't practise more than you can bear. See Chapter Two for details.

5) Other exercises

If a patient suffers osteophyte on the heel, practise more walking exercise, if on the lumbar vertebra, sleep on a bed, if on the cervical vertebra, sleep on a low pillow or sleep without it.

3. Sample Case

Ms. Xin, 49 years old, had suffered from pain in the heels for half a year, with no relief. She was all right at work, but felt pain while resting or sleeping, and could not bear to put the heels on the ground. The pain could be relieved only after massage. An X-ray showed she had osteophyte on the heels. She accepted Qigong treatment, practising mainly the Longevity Exercise. One month later, half the pain was relieved. Two months later, she felt no pain and went back to normal work. No pain was felt up to the one-year follow-up survey.

ANGITIS

Angitis is a disease characterized by the small arteries in the limbs being blocked as a result of chronic inflammation.

1. Clinical Manifestations

The main symptoms are that the patient feels numbness, coldness, tingling, swollenness and pain. It gets worse when standing and walking, and sometimes the patients become lame, experience myophagism and the limbs become thinner, or the tissues show ulceration or necrosis.

2. Qigong Treatment

1) Respiration Following the Mind Exercise

Lie on the back with a low pillow. Loosen the clothes and belt, getting into quiescence naturally. Half-close the eyes and put the arms at the sides. Breathe following the mind, making it deep, long, thin, even, stable and slow. Breathe 8 to 10 times per minute, practising 10 to 15 minutes.

2) Internal *Qi* Respiration Exercise

Lie on the back. Relax the whole body and get into quiescence. Put two pillows under the affected limb, concentrate the mind on Shanzhong, stretch out the arms and take deep breaths 3 to 6 times. Then hold the hands 2 to 3 cm above Shanzhong with one hand on the other, taking this as the beginning point to write a figure 8 around the breasts, breathing once for each 8. Write 8 50 times clockwise and 50 counter clockwise. Before finishing the exercise, stretch out the arms and take deep breaths another 3 to 6 times.

3) Qiaoqiao (Seesaw) Exercise

See the previous section of gastroptosia for details.

When practising the Qigong exercises, the patient should be relaxed, quiescent, natural, gradual and persistent, and should combine the mind with *qi* and mainly practise the quiescent exercises, with the motional ones being auxiliary. If the patient experiences ulceration or necrosis, he or she should practise the lying exercise only 3 to 4 times a day and no less than 4 hours altogether.

3. Sample Case

Mr. Zhai, 35 years old, had suffered from angitis for 5 years. His big toe and second toe on the left foot and the big toe on the right foot were amputated. His doctor had advised him to have his second and third toes on the right foot amputated but he did not consent. He turned to Qigong exercises, practising the breathing and Qiaoqiao (Seesaw) and other exercises more than 4 hours a day. One month later, the red and blue colours on his toes disappeared, the pain was relieved, with only the numbness and swollen sensation remained and he could walk. Three months later, he felt nothing wrong on his toes and went back to work. He continued to practise Qigong exercises. No relapse was found at the 5-year follow-up survey.

PERIPHERAL NEURITIS

Peripheral neuritis is also called around neuritis. It is mainly characterized by the disturbance of sensation and movement in the limbs.

1. Clinical Manifestations

The main symptoms are the disturbance of the sensation and movement of the extremities, as if wearing gloves and socks. The patient feels pain and numbness and the sensation of ants crawling on the skin, along with a weakening of the muscle tension in the hands and feet.

2. Qigong Treatment

1) Quiescent Sitting Health Cultivation Exercise.

Take the second respiration method, concentrating the mind on Dantian point. Practise 3 times a day, 30 to 60 minutes each time. See Chapter Two for details.

2) Eight Pieces of Brocade Exercise, Sinew-transforming Exercise and the Five Animals Frolic.

Choose one of the above exercises and practise 1 or 2 times a day, 30 minutes each time. See Chapter Two for details.

The Qigong exercises can promote the circulation of the blood and *qi* and have curative effect on peripheral neuritis.

CHRONIC NEPHIRITIS

Chronic nephritis, also called chronic glomerulo-nephritis, is a kind of inflammatory injury of the glomerulus. It is often found in young and middle-aged men.

1. Clinical Manifestations

The main symptoms are dropsy, protein in the urine, bloody urine, cylindraria, high blood pressure and kidney dysfunction to various degrees.

2. Qigong Treatment

1) Relaxing Exercise

Practise either the Three-line Relaxing Exercise or Relaxing Exercise. See the previous sections of hypertension and apoplexy sequelae.

2) Quiescent and Stopping Respiration Exercise

Get up at 3 to 4 o'clock, drink 300 to 400 ml of warm boiled water and relieve yourself. Then stand in open, facing the south. Hold the hands in half fists with the palms inward, relaxing the whole body and stopping all distracting thoughts—bring yourself into a state of looking but seeing nothing and listening but hearing nothing. Use the counter respiration method, inhaling through the nose while drawing back the abdomen, stretching the chest, contracting the anal sphincter and the external genital organ, licking the palate with tongue tip and concentrating the mind on Baihui. After inhaling, stop respiration for a while. Then lower the tongue, swallow the saliva in several times and, using the mind, send it to Dantian. At the same time, relax the whole body. Exhale through both nose and mouth, float the abdomen and concentrate the mind on Dantian. Repeat 7 times. After taking a little rest, repeat another 7 times. Practise one to two hours a day, but pay attention not to inhale and exhale too strongly and quickly. In particular, do not hold the breath for too long to avoid the suffocation.

3) Sky-facing Respiration Exercise

Stand with the hands on the back waist (put the Laogong points against the Shenyu points). Throw out the head and look at the sky while inhaling. Inhale air as you lean the upper body backwards about 20 to 50 degress, throwing out the chest but not holding the breath. Then make the upper body straight gradually while exhaling. Repeat 5 to 15 minutes.

4) Longevity Exercise

Choose the 1st, 3rd, 7th and 20th postures to practise. See Chapter Two for details.

3. Sample Case

According to the information provided by Shuguang Hospital in Shanghai, 13 out of 17 chronic nephritis patients who had no improvement after long-term treatment with traditional Chinese and Western medicine, got well to various degrees after practising Qigong, mainly Relaxing Exercise. They said that they were in high spirit, appetite was improved and symptoms, such as the feeling of pain and tingling in the back, were relieved. Chemical examination showed that the index of the protein urine was reduced in seven of them, and five patients' protein urine index were even reduced within 24 hours after Qigong treatment. The renal function was improved and nitroginous quantity decreased in one of them. The blood pressure was reduced in two of them.

SEXUAL IMPOTENCE

Sexual impotence refers to a man's penis not erecting or erecting without enough hardness. It is usually caused by disturbance of the controlling function of the penis erection in the cerebral cortex or spinal central nervous system. Neurasthenia, chronic backaches and excessive sex life can also cause the disease.

1. Clinical Manifestations

The patient's penis wilts or erects without enough hardness, accompanied with dizziness, vexation, uneasiness, disturbed sleep, pain in the back and knees.

2. Qigong Treatment

1) Quiescent Sitting Health Cultivation Exercises

Practise 2 to 3 times a day, 30 minutes each time. See Chapter Two for details.

2) Longevity Exercise, Eight Pieces of Brocade Exercise and the Five Animals Frolic

Choose one of the above exercises, practise 1 or 2 times a day, 15 minutes each time. See Chapter Two for details.

3) Masculine-strengthening Exercise

Practise before going to bed.

a. Sit with the legs crossed. Massage the Yongquan points on the feet with the Laogong points of the palms for 18 times, with left palm to the left foot and right palm to the right foot. Then rub and press the navel 18 times with the right hand and another 18 times with the left, then rub and press the two sides of the body with the two hands for 18 times, then massage the abdomen with the palms of the hands each for 18 times, and finally rock the shoulders up and down for 18 times. Take a rest quiescently for a moment, then swallow the saliva with force and send it to Dantian. Clench the fists with the thumbs inside, sit quiescently, calm the thoughts, regulate the breath, concentrate the mind on Dantian and count the breaths to 81 times. Then stretch the legs and sleep on the side.

b. Sit with the Yongquan point of one foot opposite to the Yongquan point of the other and rub them each other till you feel warm in the feet. Then add the abdominal respiration method, making the breath deep, slow, thin and even, making the mind and *qi* follow it. While inhaling, contract the anal sphincter and think the *qi* entering Huiyin point, through the Weilü point to Mingmen. Hold the breath for a moment, then exhale from Dantian to Huiyin. Repeat the respiration 18 times. Then do the same, but imagine the *qi* coming in from Huiyin, and up to Dantian and contract the anal sphincter. Hold the breath for a moment, then exhale it to Mingmen, and then return it to Huiyin.

c. Lie on the back and relax the whole body. Rub the testicles and groin up and down with the hands, together for 36 times. Then bend with knees. Support the testicles with the right hand rub the lower abdomen with the left hand for 36 times in a circle. Then exchange the two hands to do the same. Do this 9 times. At last support the testicles with the left hand, put the right hand on the navel and lie quiescently to cultivate the *qi* and store energy.

Choose one of the above 3 postures to practise, or practise all of them. The exercises have effect not only on sexual impotence, but also on premature ejaculation, emission, etc.

4) Expectant Point Massage

Press and rub the Guanyuan, Zhongji and Sanyinjiao points with the thumb or the middle finger each point for one minute. Then rub the penis with the two palms for 100 times.

3. Sample Case

A 30 year old male patient accepted Qigong treatment for the first time in July 1982. He had suffered from premature ejaculation for 6 to 7 years. He had a history of masturbation. His penis had not been able to erect for one year and he had no change with medical treatment. The accompanying symptoms were tiredness, backaches and vivid dreams. His pulse was faint, thin and weak. His tongue was pale and the coating of the tongue was thin and yellow. After practising Qigong exercises for 25 times, his penis could erect again, his sexual life returned to normal and his other symptoms disappeared as well.

DIABETES MELLITUS

Diabetes mellitus is a kind of systemic disease caused by a difficiency of insulin secretion which results in a disorder of the glucose's metabolism. Its incidence rate rises with age. Men are slightly more susceptible than women.

1. Clinical Manifestations

The main symptoms are diuresis, overdrinking, overeating, leanness, tiredness, dizziness and lethargy or insomnia and pain in limbs and back.

2. Qigong Treatment

There are three main kinds of treatments for diabetes mellitus. They are dietotherapy, chemotherapy, and exercise treatment. Adequate exercise is helpful to improve glucose metabolism, and prevent complications and expanding of diabetes mellitus. Qigong exercise is not only simple and convenient, but an effective way.

1) Relaxing Exercise

Practise 3 to 5 times a day, 20 to 30 minutes each time. Both the Relaxing Exercise and Three-line Relaxing Exercise will do. See the previous sections of hypertension and apoplexy sequelae for details.

2) Ball-blowing Exercise

Practise 4 to 6 times a day. See the previous sections of chronic bronchitix and pneumonectasis (the 9th posture, ball-blowing). Attention: Either of two respiration methods can be used in the exercise, thoracic and abdominal. If you take the lying posture and adopt the thoracic respiration method, do not use a pillow, put your hands under the head and concentrate the mind on Shangen point. If you adopt the abdominal respiration method, put the hands on the sides of the body, stretch the arms, lie on a pillow, relax the abdominal muscles naturally and concentrate the mind on the middle Dantian point. The distance between the ball and the mouth should be about 7 to 9 cm. Blow the ball 10 to 20 times. If it is necessary for the patient's condition, add another 50 to 100 times.

3) Heaven to Earth Exercise

Get up at about 3 to 5 o'clock in the morning. Sit with the body inclined backward slightly. Raise up one hand with the palm facing upward as high as possible. Exert all your strength to press the other hand down with the palm downward. Then exchange the hands and practise up and down in turns 36 times. Make the *qi* and the mind follow it, exhaling the waste air and inhaling the fresh. Then cultivate quiescently, tap the teeth and swallow the saliva.

4) Morning Walking Exercise

See Chapter Two for details.

5) Quiescent Sitting Health Cultivation Exercise and Relaxed Quiescent Recumbent Exercise.

Practise 2 to 3 times a day, 30 to 60 minutes each time. Choose one of them to practise. See Chapter Two for details.

6) Health Cultivation Massage

Get up early to practise every day and massage the Shenyu point on the waist 36 to 72 times after the exercise.

3. Sample Case

Mr. Zhang, 65 years old, had suffered from thirst, overeating and diuresis, accompanied with weakness and numbness on the lower limbs, for more than two years. Examination showed that his blood sugar was 280 mg, the glucose in urine was a strongly positive reaction with 4 pluses. He was diagnosed as having diabetes mellitus. At the beginning of the medical treatment, through control of the diet, the symptoms were relieved and the blood sugar decreased, but the symptoms recurred occasionally. A year later, he turnd to Qigong treatment. After two months practise, his symptoms were relieved and the blood sugar decreased to 160 mg, while the glucose urine was two pluses. His symptoms disappered basically and the blood sugar was controlled at the normal level after continuing Qigong exercises for 4 months. One year later, he has been released of some of his dietary limitations and the curative effect was still stable.

PROSTATOMEGALY

Prostatomegaly is a common disease in old men. It is probably related to overactive sexual life, bladder hyperemia and disorder of sexual hormone balance.

1. Clinical Manifestations

The main symptoms are pollakiuria, urgency of urination, urodynia, urine incontinence, dysuria, even acute retention of urine. The serious patient may have hematuria.

2. Qigong Treatment

1) Longevity Exercise

Practise 1 or 2 times a day, about 30 minutes each time. See Chapter Two for details.

2) Lifting *Qi* Exercise

Practise 3 to 5 times a day. See the previous section of proctoptosis for details.

3) Internal *Qi* Respiration Exercise

Practise 3 to 5 times a day, 10 minutes each time. See the previous section of angitis for details.

4) Respiration Following the Mind Exercise

Practise 3 to 5 times a day, 10 minutes each time. See the previous section of angitis.

5) Hip-raising Exercise

a. Lie on the back with the legs bent and put the shanks vertically on the bed. With the shoulders and the feet as the supporting points, raise the hips, breathe deeply and contract the anal sphincter for 3 to 5 seconds. Then lower the hips in order to strengthen the rocking force, meanwhile relaxing the whole body and breathing deeply. Repeat 20 to 50 times.

b. Lie on the back, raise the hips high and inhale deeply. Then hold the breath and twist the hips with force from the right to the left. Then lower the hips and breathe deeply. Repeat 10 to 20 times.

6) Expectant Point Massage

a. Rub and massage the lower abdomen 20 to 30 times. Press and massage the Qihai, Guanyuan, Zhongji, Sanyinjiao and Yinlingquan points for one minute each to make them gain *qi*.

b. Rub the lower abdomen and lumbosacral area 100 times each.

7) Other supplementary treatments

a. Sunbath: You can take any posture as long as the sunlight shines on the perineum directly and you feel warm in the hips. Have sunbath for 5 minutes each day, gradually prolonging the time. The best time for sunbath is 8 to 10 a.m. and from 2 to 4 p.m, when there are relatively more ultraviolet rays. The goal of the exercise is to enhance the blood circulation of the prostate.

b. Swimming: You can take any style of swimming. The water temperature should be at about 25°C. Swim once a day or once every other day, 20 to 30 minutes each time. The goal of the exercise is to get rid of the hyperemia of the pelvic organs.

3. Sample Case

Mr. Zhang, 39 years old, had suffered from pollakiuria, dizziness, white liquid flowing from the urethra after urination, impotence, tightness in the perineum and occasional chest distress and insomnia for 6 years. After examinations in several hospitals, he was diagnosed as having prostatomegaly. His condition turned better after taking some Western and traditional Chinese medicine, but the symptoms recurred later with dysuria. Hoping to be cured completely, he turned to Qigong treatment, practising Qigong exercises indoors everyday. Meanwhile he took swims and had sunbath. The symptoms disappeared completely in half a year. The examination and test results showed that the prostatic node had disappeared and the size of the prostate had been reduced from the size of an egg to the size of a chestnut, and his prostatic smear and culture all showed negative reaction. Now he is continuing practising the Qigong exercises in his sparetime so as to consolidate the curative effect.

VARICOCELE

Varicocele is a disease with symptoms of lumbago and dragging sensation in the scrotum, usually caused by funicular varicostion. It may affect the patient's sexual function and is often found in middle-aged and old men.

1. Clinical Manifestations

The patient feels dragging sensation and pain in the scrotum when walking and standing, the pain even spreading to the waist (mostly on the left). The spermatic cord is hypertrophic. There are some irregular soft lumps in the scrotum with the small ends upward and the bases covering the patient's testicle. The scrotum swells down over the glans penis 2 to 4 cm.

2. Qigong Treatment

1) Sitting and Lying Exercise

Sit upright or with the legs crossed and get into quiescence naturally. Following the mind, make the breaths deep, long, thin, even, steady and slow. Breathe 8 to 10 times per minute, practising 30 minutes each time. You can also take the supine lying posture. When lying, put the scrotum on the thighs and put the arms beside the body or beside the head. Get into quiescence and regulate the breath as in the sitting practise. Practise twice a day, in the morning and evening, 10 to 15 minutes each time.

2) Qiaoqiao (Seesaw) Exercise

See the previous section of gastroptosia for details.

3) Self-massage Exercise

Put the legs sidewards with the knees bent. Support the scrotum with one hand and rub it or raise and shake it with the other. Practise twice a day, in the morning and evening, 10 to 15 minutes each time.

4) Swimming Exercise

Swim mainly in the backstroke style, using the breast stroke and butterfly stroke as auxiliary means. The patient should maintain unobstruction of the stool, relieve the lower abdomen from all pressure and avoid excessive fatigue, standing for long periods, walking and jogging.

3. Sample Case

Mr. Wang, 38 years old, had suffered from the dragging sensation in the scrotum, lumbago, backaches, premature ejaculation, emission, insomnia and discomfort when walking for 6 years. He was diagnosed as having left varicocele after examination. He took Qigong treatment, practising the sitting and lying, Qiaoqiao, and self-massage exercises in the morning and evening. He also had a cold waterbath, sunbath and airbath and wore tight underwear. Two years later, his left scrotum rose up from 4 cm below the glans penis to 3 cm above it, as high as the right one, and was no longer swollen. The soft lump in the scrotum disappeared. No abnormal phenomenon was found in the one-year follow-up survey. Now he is still practising the Qigong exercises in order to consolidate the curative effect.

ALOPECIA AREATA

The cause of the disease is still unknown. Usually one part or several parts of the patient's hair fall out overnight. Sometimes the bald area is small, and sometimes is big. The patients suffer much from this.

1. Clinical Manifestations

It often occurs suddenly at night, to be found the next day. The bald parts are smooth, round or elliptical, small or big. The roots of the hair can't be found. There is neither inflammation nor unusual sensation.

2. Qigong Treatment

1) Three Inhalings and Three Exhalings Exercise

Take either a sitting or lying posture. If you take the supine lying posture, stretch the arms along the head, half-close the eyes, relax and get into quiescence for 20 seconds. Inhale 3 times continously, then exhaling 3 times. Don't hold breath during respiration. Practise 30 minutes each time. If you practise indoors, you should open the windows. If outdoors, you should choose a place with fresh air. If you choose the sitting posture, use the same respiration method, putting the hands on the knees.

2) Longevity Exercise

Practise the 1st and 20th postures 2 to 3 times a day, 15 to 30 minutes each time. See Chapter Two for details.

3. Sample Case

Mr. Zhang, 38 yesrs old, a part of his hair on the back of his head fell off suddenly overnight. The skin of the part was smooth, without the marks of hair roots or inflammation. He had no improvement with treatment with ginger roots and trichogen. He turned to Qigong treatment. A Qigong master advised him to practise Up-and-Down Respiration-adjusting Exercise. One month later, some thin and yellow hair grew. Two months later, some black hair appeared. After three months, black hair had grown out of the whole bald area.

VITILIGO

Vitiligo is a disease characterized by leukasmus on the skin, but with no uncomfortable sensation. It can be found in people at any age, but male patients are slightly more susceptible.

1. Clinical Manifestations

The patient experiences leukasmus on the skin. The leukasmus may be large or small, in round, elliptical or irregular shape. Inside the leukasmus the hair becomes white encircled with a dark pigment bend. Sometimes pigmentation appears in the leukasmus. The amount of the leukasmus is uncertain, sometimes occurring over the whole body, but usually the patient has no uncomfortable sensation.

2. Qigong Treatment

1) Longevity Exercise

This is main exercise for treating vitiligo. Practise 2 to 3 times a day, 30 minutes each time. See Chapter Two for details.

2) Three 8-shape *Qi* Drivng Cultivation Exercise

Practise 2 to 3 times a day. See the previous section of chronic bronchitis and emphysema for details.

3) Take sunbath, waterbath and airbath as the auxiliary means to the Qigong treatment. Properly coordinate with oral medicine, Chinese herbal medicine for external application, magnetoelectric treatment, and so on. The patient should stop smoking and drinking, have a balanced diet, eat food which is rich in calcium, copper and iron and foods rich in melanin, such as black soya beans and black sesame.

The Long-term experience has proved that comprehensive Qigong treatment has an ideal effect on the disease.

3. Sample Case

Min, a young man of 18 years old, had suffered from vitiligo on the back of his head for 3 years. He was treated in several hospitals, but with no effect. On the contrary, the leukasmus enlarged and his hair turned white. When he turned to Qigong treatment, his condition took a favourable turn. He was cured in six months. No relapse in the old area and no new leukasmus were found in the three-year follow-up survey.

CHRONIC PELVIC INFLAMMATION

Chronic pelvic inflammation affects organs in the pelvic cavity (including the oviducts, ovarium and pelvic connective tissue) caused by bacterial infection. It may attack repeatedly.

1. Clinical Manifestations

The main symptoms are pain in the lower abdomen, abdominal distension, lumbago and increased leucorrhoea. Sometimes it is accompanied with dizziness, headaches, chest distress, weariness, insomnia, constipation, menoxenia and so on.

2. Qigong Treatment

1) Quiescent Sitting Health Cultivation Exercise or Relaxed and Quiescent Recumbent Lying Exercise

Practise 2 or 3 times a day, 30 minutes each time. See Chapter Two for details.

2) Relaxing Exercise

You can choose either the Relaxing Exercise or the Three-line Relaxing Exercise. Practise 2 or 3 times a day, 30 minutes each time. See the previous sections of hypertension and apoplexy sequelae.

3) Sinew-transforming Exercise, Eight Pieces of Brocade Exercise and Longevity Exercise

Practise 1 or 2 times a day, 15 minutes each time. See Chapter Two for details.

4) Expectant Point Massage

Pinch the lower abdomen 20 to 30 times. Then press the Daju, Xuehai and

Sanyinjiao points, each for one minute. Do this twice a day.

3. Sample Case

Ms. Zhang, 57 years old, had experienced childbirth 3 times, and now has two children. The last birth was in 1959. She suffered from acute appendicitis and had an operation in 1961. In 1967, she felt discomfort in the lower abdomen, and pain before and after menses, accompanied with lumbago. Her menses were irregular and profuse with dark colour. She was diagnosed as having pelvic inflammation. In 1977, the pain in her lower abdomen and lumbago became severe, and she was diagnosed as having chronic pelvic inflammation. She turned to comprehensive Qigong treatment. Three months later her symptoms were improved. She continued with the exercises and her condition remained stable.

METROPTOSIS

Metroptosis is characterized by the position of the womb being lower than normal. It happens just because the ligaments supporting the womb become loose, usually caused by the increased pressure on the abdomen resulting from excessive childbirth, physical labour too soon after childbirth, standing for long periods, and chronic coughing.

1. Clinical Manifestations

The patient feels something tenesmus in the pudenda. The less serious patients may feel lumbago and tenesmus in the lower abdomen only. In relatively serious cases, the cervix of the womb may drop out of the vagina entrance. In serious cases, the cervix and the whole womb may drop out, the symptoms usually being accompanied by frequency of micturition and dysuria.

2. Qigong Treatment

1) Relaxed and Quiescent Recumbent Exercise

Take the 1st respiration method and concentrate the mind on the Dantian or Huiyin point. Practise 2 to 4 times a day, 40 minutes each time. See Chapter Two for details.

2) Lifting *Qi* Exercise

Practise 3 to 5 times a day, 5 minutes each time. See the previous section of proctoptosis.

3) Longevity Exercise, Buddha's Guardians' Exercise and Eight Pieces of Brocade Exercise.

Choose one of the above exercises as the auxiliary means to the quiescent exercise. Practise once or twice a day, 15 minutes each time. See Chapter Two for details.

4) Masculine-strengthening Exercise

Practise the 2nd posture. See the previous section of sexual impotence.

5) Expectant Point Massage

a. Massage the lower abdomen with the palm in a circle 40 to 50 times, then pinch the muscles on the lower abdomen 20 to 30 times.

b. Knead the Shenyu points with the palms for 72 times, then press the Sanyinjiao, Xuehai and Huiyin points each for one minute.

MENOPAUSAL SYNDROME

Menopausal syndrome refers to a series of symptoms of vegetative nervous function disorder caused by the declined ovary function during the period of women's amenia menischesis. The patient may also have a series of symptoms of visceral function disorder.

1. Clinical Manifestations

The main symptoms are mental stress, mood undulation, hypomesis, distraction, diverting, insomnia, over-dream, lassitude, weariness, dizziness, shortness of breath, hectic fever, sweating, blood pressure undulation and menses disorder.

2. Qigong Treatment

The patient can choose the Qigong exercises according to her own symptoms. For instance, if the patient has high blood pressure or obvious nervous system symptoms, she should choose the relaxing exercise to adjust the nervous system. See the previous section of hypertension for details.

If the patient is thin and weak and has disturbance in the digestive system, she should choose the Relaxed and Quiescent Recumbent Exercise with the second respiration method to improve the appetite, prompt digestion and strengthen the constitution. She can also choose some motional exercises to combine with the quiescent ones, such as the Eight Pieces of Brocade Exercise, Longevity Exercise and Sinew-transforming Exercise.

If the patient has hectic fever, she should choose to practise the inhaling exercises, such as the first respiration method in the Quiescent Sitting Health Cultivation Exercise, to alleviate or remove the symptoms through stimulating sympathetic nerve's excitation.

In addition, besides the above exercises, the patients can also practise the massage cultivation exercises, such as knocking the ears, kneading the waist and Yongguan points, as the auxiliary means. Practise the above exercises 2 or 3 times a day, 50 minutes each time.

DYSMENORRHEA

Dysmenorrhea is a disease involving paroxysmal pain in the lower abdomen before, during or after menses. It usually relates to local genital pathologic changes, hypoplasia of the uterus, stenosis of the cervix, metropolypus, inflammation, mental stress and catching cold.

1. Clinical Manifestations

Before or during menses, the patient has pain in the lower abdomen, lumbago, distending pain in both of the breasts and menses hindrance. The serious patient may have sharp pain, nausea, vomiting, dizziness and a cold feeling in the hands and feet. The pain disappears naturally after the menses period.

2. Qigong Treatment

In general, Qigong treatment is only suitable to the primary dysmenorrhea and to the people who have no organic pathologic changes in the genital organ and functional dysmenorrhea. The primary dysmenorrhea often occur in unmarried women or young women who have never been pregnant.

1) Relaxing Exercise

Choose either the Relaxing Exercises or the Three-line Relaxing Exercise. Practise 3 to 4 times a day, 30 minutes each time. See the previous sections of hypertension and apoplexy sequelae for details.

2) Sinew-transforming Exercise and Longevity Exercise

Practise 1 or 2 times a day, 15 to 20 minutes each time. See Chapter Two for details.

3) Air Bicycle-riding Exercise

Lie on the back and lift the legs high into the air, bend and stretch the hipjoint and knees in turn as if riding a bicycle (Fig. 93-1) dozens of times. Rest for a while. Then stretch the legs straight. Raise one leg at an angle of about 45 degrees with an abduction of about 20 degrees. Taking the hip joint as the axis, move the leg in a circle from small to large (Fig. 93-2). Repeat 10 to 50 times.

4) Expectant Point Massage

Knead the lower abdomen with the palm 20 to 30 times. Massage the lumbosacral part and internal thighs 20 to 30 times respectively. Then press the Xuehai, Sanyinjiao, Guanyuan and Laogong points one minute each. Practise this every morning and evening.

MENSTRUAL DISORDER

Menstrual disorder is characterized by abnormalities of period, amount, colour and the property of the menstruation.

1. Clinical Manifestations

The main symptoms are advanced or delayed menses, irregular menses, menorrheal, hypomenorrhea and prolonged menses, etc.

2. Qigong Treatment

1)Relaxing Exercise

Choose either the Three-line Relaxing Exercise or the Relaxing Exercise.

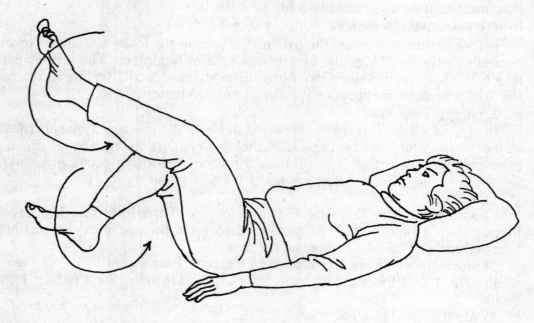

Fig. 93-1

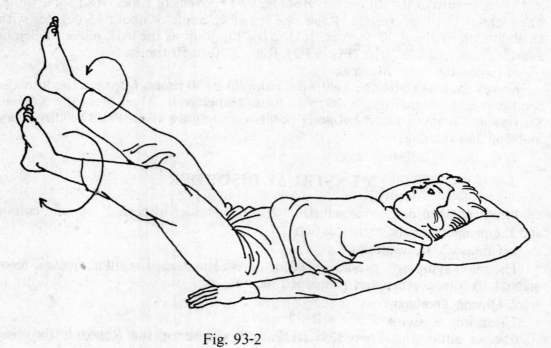

Fig. 93-2

Practise 2 to 3 times a day, 30 minutes each time. See the previous sections of hypertension and the apoplexy sequelae for details.

2) Modulating and Recuperating Exercise

Sit straight on the front of a stool or chair with the feet a shoulder width apart on the floor. Bend the knees in 90 degrees, put the right hand on the navel with the internal Laogong point against it, put the left hand on the right one with the internal Laogong against the right's external Laogong point. Close the eyes and mouth slightly, with the tongue touching the palate. Relax the whole body, dismiss all the disturbing thoughts and regulate the breath. When inhaling, draw back the abdomen and contract the anal sphincter so as to tense the perinium. Then, following the mind, move the *qi* up from Huiyin to Dantian and accumulate it there. When exhaling, relax the anus and abdomen. Repeat the respiration like this for 30 minutes, then rub the face gently with the hands as if washing the face, 5 to 7 times. Then stand up and stop the exercise.

3. Sample Case

A 24-year-old married woman had been bleeding continually since the intrauterine ring was fitted, and there had not been improvement even after treatment in hospital. A month later, she turned to Qigong treatment. The out-patient department taught her to practise the Modulating and Recuperating Exercise. Half an hour later, the bleeding had diminished. After practising the exercise for two days—twice a day in the morning and evening, 30 minutes each time—the bleeding had stopped completely. The next month her menses was normal as expected and cleared up naturally in 6 days. A half-year follow-up survey showed that the period and amount of her menses had been normal since.

DYSFUNCTIONAL UTERINE BLEEDING

Dysfunctional uterine bleeding is a kind of disease with irregular or excessive vaginal bleeding caused by the dysfunction of the ovaries.

1. Clinical Manifestations

The main symptoms are irregular or excessive vaginal bleeding after menses, often complicated with vertigo, dizziness, lumbago, tiredness, dysphoria with a smothery sensation.

2. Qigong Treatment

1) Relaxing Exercise

Choose either the Three-line Relaxing Exercise or the Relaxing Exercise. Practise 3 times a day, 20 minutes each time. See the previous sections of hypertension and apoplexy sequelae.

2) Sitting or Lying Respiration Exercise

Lie, or sit with the knees crossed, relax in quiescence, respirate naturally and concentrate the mind on Shanzhong point. Practise 3 to 5 times a day, 30 minutes each time. See the previous sections of hypertention and apoplexy sequelae for details.

3) Three 8-shape *Qi* Driving Cultivation Exercise

Practise 2 to 3 times a day, 30 minutes each time. See the previous section of chronic bronchitis and emphysema.

4) Expectant Points Massage

a. Knead the lower abdomen with the palm for 20 to 30 times.

b. Massage the lumbosacral region and the internal thighs for 20 to 30 times respectively. Repeat more on the aching points.

c. Press the Quchi, Yanglingquan, Sanyinjiao and Xuehai points for one minute each.

MYOPIA

Myopia is a disease caused by ametropia. It is common in primary and middle-school students. Mostly it results from long-term improper use of the eyes, such as working at a short distance, reading in dim light or in an incorrect posture, or is due to genetic factors.

1. Clinical Manifestations

The patient can see things close up but unclear at a distance.

2. Qigong Treatment

1) Three 8-shape *Qi* Driving Cultivation Exercise

Practise 3 times a day, 30 minutes each time. See the previous section of chronic bronchitis and emphysema.

2) Relaxing Exercise

Relax the eyes, breathe naturally, and concentrate the mind on Dantian. See the previous sections of hypertension and apoplexy sequelae.

3) Laogong Eye-activating Exercise

Hold the palms opposite to each other at a distance of 12 inches. When you feel the repulsive force, put the Laogong points on the eyes, and move the hands clockwise and counterclockwise 18 times each. Close the eyes for a moment, then open them and look at a distant object for 1 to 2 minutes. Repeat several times a day.

4) Nose-watching Exercise

Keep quiescent, breathe naturally and concentrate the mind. Put the index fingers on the nose tip with the thumbs touching the lower jaw slightly and the other fingers closed naturally. Gaze upon the index fingers for 2 to 3 seconds, then look at a small target 20 metres away, focussing on it as clearly as possible. Then withdraw the sight and look at the nose tip again. Repeat 3 to 5 times, then rest for a minute and do the same again. Do 3 sequences.

5) Expectant Point Massage

a. Pressing and rubbing the Jingming points. Close the eyes, press the two thumbs on the Jingming points, press and squeeze the base of the nose—first pressing downward then squeezing upward. Repeat like this 32 times.

b. Pressing the Taiyang points and rubbing the rims of the eyes. Rub the Zanzhu, Yuyao, Sizhukong, Tongziliao and Chengqi points first. Press the Taiyang points with the pad of the thumb and the other fingers twisted. Rub the rims of the eyes with the internal side of the second segment of the index fingers from inside to outside, first the upper rims then the lower ones. Then press the Taiyang points with the pads of the thumbs for the same period of time. Repeat 4 times.

c. Pressing and rubbing the Sibai points. Do not move the fingers away from the skin. The range of the rubbing should not be too large. Repeat 32 times.

d. Pressing and rubbing the Fengchi points. Close the index and middle fingers and rub the Fengchi points with them 32 times.

e. Dry face washing. Close the four fingers, push them from the wings of the nose upward along the bridge of the nose till reaching the forehead. Then pull the hands downward along the frontal bones and the Taiyang points. Repeat 4 times.

All the exercises mentioned above should be practised once every morning and evening.

6) Longevity Exercise

Choose the 1st and 2nd postures or the whole exercise. Practise 1 or 2 times a day, 30 to 45 minutes each time. See Chapter Two for details.

7) Correct all the bad habits when using the eyes.

3. Sample Case

Chu, a girl of 18 years old, had been nearsighted for 3 years with a vision of 0.3 for the left eye and 0.2 for the right, and wore a pair of glasses of 800 degrees negative. She practised Three 8-shape *Qi* Driving Cultivation Exercise every morning, evening and break-time, and practised Longevity Exercise every morning. Half a year later, her sight was improved, her glasses were decreased to 460 degrees negative and her vision becoming 0.6 for the left eye and 0.5 for the right. After practising Qigong exercises for another half a year, she didn't need her glasses and recovered vision of 1.2 for each eye.

SENILE CATARACTS

Cataracts are a common eye disease characterized by opacity of the capsule or fibre of the lens. It is a disease which can cause blindness and it is common in old people.

1. Clinical Manifestations

The main symptoms are that the patient's vision decreases gradually. In dim places the vision becomes worse. The symptoms are often accompanied by vertigo and limb weakness.

2. Qigong Treatment

Qigong exercises have some curative effect on the disease and can be used to treat the early patients.

1) Kidney-strengthening Exercise

Stand and collect the *qi* into the lower abdomen. Turn the upper body to the right, meanwhile, following the left hand, move the *qi* to the back along the waist. When turning the upper body to the left, press the left hand on the back of the waist and the right hand on the lower abdomen. Then turn the upper body to the right, press the left hand on the lower abdomen and the right hand on the back of the waist. After repeating 9 times, put the right hand on the lower abdomen and turn the body upright. Then, following the two hands, drive the *qi* backward along the sides of the body and lean forward. When the hands reach the back of the waist, return them to the lower abdomen again, leaning the body backward. After repeating 9 times, put the two hands on Dantian, one above the other and rub it gently. Keep the hands on the lower abdomen for a moment, then stop the exercise.

2) Three 8-shape *Qi* Driving Cultivation Exercise

Practise 2 to 3 times a day, 30 minutes each time. See the previous sections of chronic bronchitis and emphysema for details.

3) Expectant Point Massage

a. Calm the mind, sit in quiescence, close the eyes and concentrate the mind on Yintang. Breathe naturally for 7 times. Gradually move the mind to the centres of the eyeballs and keep it there for about 3 minutes.

b. Clench the hands slightly, rub the thumbs till you feel warm, then rub the rims of the eyes with the thumbs gently clockwise and inhale at the same time, then counterclockwise and exhale.

c. Clench the hands slightly, rub the thumbs till you feel warm, then rub the superciliary ridge. At the same time, sway the head to the left and the right in coordination with the hands. The movement should be gentle and slow. Inhale when the head sways to the left, and exhale when to the right. Repeat 18 times.

d. Put the pads of the thumbs on the Zanzhu points and press them, first gently then little by little, forcefully. When pressing, inhale and count to 18 in the mind; when loosening the hands, exhale and count to 18 again.

e. Put the pads of the thumbs on the Yuyao points. Press at first, then massage. When pressing, inhale and count to 18 in the mind. When rubbing, exhale and count to 18 again.

f. Bend the thumbs and index fingers as bows. Press the Yangbai points with the index fingers and Yuwei points with the thumbs simultanously. First press and inhale, then massage and exhale. Repeat 18 times.

g. First push, then pinch the Jingming points 18 times. Inhale when pushing, and exhale when pinching.

h. First pinch, then rub the Chengqi points 18 times. Inhale when pinching, and exhale when rubbing.

i. Press and rub the Sibai points 18 times. Inhale when pressing, and exhale when rubbing.

j. Press the Juliao points 18 times. Inhale when pressing, and exhale when loosening the fingers.

k. Turning the eyes. Close the eyes, calm the mind, and turn the eyeball to the right and left each 14 times. Inhale when turning to the left and exhale when turning to the right. Then stop the turning for a moment, open the eyes suddenly and gaze upon a point in front for about half a minute.

l. Rub the Taiyang points gently with the pads of the thumbs. Rub the palms warm, then dry wash the face with the hands moving from the Chengjiang point under the lips upward along the nose to the Baihui point, then passing the back of the head, the neck and the chin, and back to the Chengjiang point again. Repeat 36 times, then stop.

3. Sample Case

Mr. Li suffered from eye disease from age of 7, gradually developing cataracts over two years. He learned the point-pressing and massage exercise from a Qigong master when he was 16. After a year's practising, the disease never attacked again. He stopped practising the exercise at middle age. He had more severe cataracts in his fifties, and could not see clearly. In an operation, the pupil of the right eye was injured, while the cataract of the left eye remained unremoved. His vision decreased and the complication of inflammation occurred in the eyes. Having no improvement with medical treatment, he turned to Qigong treatment again. Half a year later, the inflammation disappeared, and a year later, his vision increased from 0.1 and 0.08 to 0.8 and 0.4 for left and right eye respectively. Six years later, his vision increased to 1.2 for the left eye and 0.8 for the right. and he was able to read even in the evening.

GLAUCOMA

Glaucoma is a eye disease caused by high pressure in the eyes, the narrowness of the anterior chambers and the hindered dischargement of the aqueous humor.

1. Clinical Manifestations

Clinically, glaucoma can be divided into acute and chronic types. When congestive glaucoma results in an acute attack, the patient may suffer severe headaches, nausea, iridization and decreased vision. Congestive ciliary body, corneal opacity, platycoria and high eye pressure can be found upon examination. Simple glaucoma attacks slowly without typical symptoms and usually is found in the late stage.

2. Qigong Treatment

1) Three-line Relaxing Exercise

Take walking, standing, sitting, or lying posture. Concentrate the mind on Taichong or Yongquan point. At the beginning, it is better to practise in the standing or sitting posture. Practise 3 times a day, 30 minutes each time, After becoming skilled, you can practise it at any time and in any posture. See the previous section of apoplexy sequelae.

2) Three 8-shape *Qi* Driving Cultivation Exercise

Practise 3 times a day, 30 minutes each time. See the previous section of chronic bronchitis and emphysema.

3) Eye Exercise

Stand with the palms downward. Relax the whole body and keep quiescent for 1 to 2 minutes. Following the mind move the *qi* from Baihui to Meizhong (the central part between the eyebrows), then separate it into two branches and move the *qi* around the rims of the eyes, at first shallow then deep and gradually making the *qi* sensable in two balls as big as table-tennis around the eyes. Following the mind, move the *qi* in a circle 7 times, then back to the Meizhong and Baihui points. Repeat the above exercise 7 times, then recite "Xu" 7 times before finishing the exercise.

3. Sample Case

A patient from Beijing suffered from primary simple glaucoma, with the eye pressure index of 29 on the left and 28 on the right and decreased vision. After practising Qigong exercises for 3 months, he felt the symptoms were obviously relieved. Six months later, his eye pressure index was decreased to 20 on the left and 18 on the right, and he had regained his vision.

ELECTRIC OPHTHALMIA

Electric ophthalmia is common radiation eye burn. It is usually caused by exposure to strong violet rays, with the symptoms often appearing 6 to 7 hours after being radiated.

1. Clinical Manifestations

Acute type: The patient experiences hyperaemia, photophobia, pain, shedding tears, and sometimes headaches and nausea. Usually the patient is unable to work.

Chronic type: The typical patient has engaged in cutting and welding with electric arc torch for a long time, and may experience photophobia and conjutive hyperaemia but can still work.

2. Qigong Treatment

1) Three 8-shape *Qi* Driving Cultivation Exercise

Practise in the spare time in the morning and evening. See the previous section of chronic bronchitis and emphysema for details.

2) Longevity Exercise

Practise the 1st and 2nd postures as the auxiliary to the Three 8-shape *Qi*

Driving Cultivation Exercise, 1 to 2 times a day, 15 to 20 minutes each time. See chapter Two for details.

3. Sample Case

Mr. Yue, 40 years old, suffered from electric ophthalmia because of his carelessness in working. He could not open his eyes. He shed tears continually, had pain in eyes, and headaches and could not go on working. He stopped shedding tears and could open his eyes after he practised the Three 8-shape *Qi* Driving Cultivation Exercise two times. Though he still felt pain in the eyes, it was much relieved. The next day he worked as usual, practising Qigong in the spare time. He recovered in three days.

MENIERE'S SYNDROME

Meniere's syndrome, also called auditory vertigo syndrome, is a severe disease caused by the oedema of the inner ear. It mainly occurs in the people at the ages of 30 to 60.

1. Clinical Manifestations

The patient falls ill suddenly, feels rotation, tinnitus, eyeball tremors, often accompanied with vomiting, pale face and cold sweating. The lasting period of the attack may be long or short. Usually the patient recovers in a few hours or a few days.

2. Qigong Treatment

1) Three 8-shape *Qi* Driving Cultivation Exercise

Practise 3 times a day, 30 minutes each time. See the previous section of chronic bronchitis and emphysema for details.

2) Relaxed and Quiescent Recumbent Exercise

Take the second respiration method and concentrate the mind on Dantian. See Chapter Two for details.

3) Expectant Point Massage

a. Lift and pull the ear roots several times with the thumbs and the index fingers, then rub the areas around the ears 20 to 30 times with the fingers.

b. Push and massage the head and waist 20 to 30 times with the palms.

c. Press the pain points on the inner side of the shanks 20 to 30 times.

d. Press the Yangchi, Mangyu, and Taixi points for one minute each.

Practise the above point-pressing and massage exercise once every morning and evening.

LARYNGOPHARYNGITIS

Laryngopharyngitis is a common disease in the department of eye, ear, nose and throat. It is often caused by bacterial or viral infections or by breathing in or eating irritating substances frequently.

1. Clinical Manifestations

The patient's throat appears red, swollen, hyperaemia, and there is pain. Pain is more obvious while swallowing. It is often accompanied with dry coughing and phlegm, occasionally with nausea and hoarseness.

2. Qigong Treatment

1) Three-line Relaxing Exercise

Stand or sit and relax along the three lines, concentrate the mind on Lieque while inhaling, and on Zhaohai while exhaling. Practise 3 times a day, 20 minutes each time. See the previous section of apoplexy sequelae.

2) The Five Animals Frolic

Practise the tiger and the bear frolics as the main exercise, 1 or 2 times a day, 10 to 20 minutes each time. See Chapter Two for details.

3) Three 8-shape *Qi* Driving Cultivation Exercise

Practise 1 or 2 times a day, 30 minutes each time. See previous section of chronic bronchitis and emphysema for details.

4) Health Cultivation Massage

Practise the licking the palate and swallowing the saliva methods. See Chapter Two for details.

5) Expectant Point Massage

Rub the two sides of the throat 20 to 30 times with the thumb, index and middle finger. Pinch the skin of the throat area 20 to 30 times till the local skin turns red and you feel hot in the throat. Then press Yifeng, Tiantu and Hegu points one minute each. Practise twice a day.

3. Sample Case

Ms. Zhang, had suffered from chronic pharyngitis for many years. She often felt uncomfortable, dry and itchy in the pharynx. The symptoms were worse and she felt severe pain when swallowing saliva and food, and whenever she had infections in the upper respiratory passage or caught a cold. She accepted medical treatment but had no improvement. Then she turned to Qigong exercises. One week later, her pharynx felt moist, smooth, painless and there was no uncomfortable sensation.

CHRONIC RHINOPATHY

Chronic rhinopathy is nose disease including chronic simple rhinitis, chronic thick rhinitis and chronic and festering nasal sinusitis, usually caused by catching cold, sysmetic diseases, or an irritative environment. These factors may attack each other and make it difficult to recover from the disease.

1. Clinical Manifestations

Chronic simple rhinitis is a kind of nasal obstruction in the two nasal cavities.

The nasal obstruction for chronic hyertrophic rhinitis is more severe, with more nasal discharge of mucus or festering. The symptoms of chronic nasal sinusitis are similar to the former, but the amount of the nasal discharge is greater and in a smell of stench, often accompanied with headache and dizziness.

2. Qigong Treatment

1) Three 8-shape *Qi* Driving Cultivation Exercise

Practise 2 or 3 times a day, 30 minutes each time. See the previous section of chronic bronchitis and emphysema.

2) Standing Straight Like a Stake Cultivation Exercise

Breathe naturally, concentrating the mind on Yongquan point. Practise twice a day 30 minutes each time. See Chapter Two for details.

3) Expectant Point Massage

Rub and pinch the two wings of the nose 20 to 30 times with the thumb, index and middle fingers. Press the Bitong, Shousanli, Hegu, Chengqi, Sibai and Mei-zhong points each for one minute. Practise 3 times a day.

3. Sample Case

Qiao had suffered from rhinitis more than 20 years. At the beginning, the nasal obstruction occurred with a cold. Later, the lower conchas became hypertrophied and ventilation was more difficult. He experienced nasal obstruction, headaches and tighness of breath, and it was difficult for him to fall asleep. His nose was clear for only four hours after using nose drops. Then he turned to Qigong treatment. He recovered after practising Qigong exercises for more than a year, and has not had a lapse since.

CHRONIC TYMPANITIS

Chronic tympanitis is a common disease which often develops from the failure of acute tympanitis treatment or incorrect treatment.

1. Clinical Manifestations

The main symptoms are perforation of the tympanic membrane of long-term, frequent or repeated festering in the ear, accompanied with double hearing, tinnitus, headaches and dizziness.

2. Qigong Treatment

1) Standing Straight Like a Stake Cultivation Exercise

Breathe naturally and concentrate the mind on Dantian and the affected ear. Practise twice a day, 20 minutes each time. See Chapter Two for details.

2) Ear Massage to Strengthen Health

Practise twice a day, 10 minutes each time. See Chapter Two for details.

3) Three 8-shape *Qi* Driving Cultivation Exercise

Practise twice a day, 30 minutes each time. See the previous section of chronic bronchitis and emphysema.

4) Longevity Exercise, Taiji Boxing, and other exercises

Practise the exercises according to the patient's constitution.

3. Sample Case

A patient from Sichuan Province had suffered from chronic tympanitis for more than 30 years. The disease recurring each time he caught a cold. Then he turned to Qigong treatment, mainly practising Standing Straight Like a Stake Cultivation Exercise, and using the massage and kneading methods as the auxiliary means. One week later, he felt better. His symptoms never recurred and his hearing was improved after practising Qigong exercises for two more months.

Chapter Four
THE ACCESSORY THERAPEUTIC METHOD OF QIGONG FOR CARCINOSIS

Carcinosis is a malignant tumour. Although at present there are therapeutic treatment methods being used, a cure is by no means guaranteed. In recent years, this disease has been treated with an integration of traditional Chinese medicine and Western medicine. When Qigong is introduced as an accessory, the therapeutic effect is often enhanced. In some cases, the symptoms are relieved, and the development of the disease is controlled so that the survival time is prolonged. In other cases, the patients are cured. This shows the heartening trend of treating cancer with Qigong. Qigong therapy does not kill normal cells, as does chemotherapy and radiotherapy which are used to kill the cancer cells, and enhance the autoimmune system, it can also help patients to regulate themselves and create an optimum external and internal environment for recovery from the disease.

As a method for the prevention and treatment of cancers, Qigong should work together with other therapeutic steps, including surgery, chemotherapy, radiotherapy, and simple and specific prescriptions, for well-rounded treatment. Generally, the patient should practise Qigong for 4 hours a day, health conditions permitting. When there is a will and perseverance, good results will be obtained.

NASOPHARYNGEAL CARCINOMA

Nasopharyngeal carcinoma is a malignant tumour mostly found in the nasopharyngeal region of the body. It often occurs in adult patients of 30 to 50 years old.

1. Clinical Manifestations
Stuffy nose, epistaxis, tinnitus, headaches, deviation of the eyes and mouth, blepharoptosis, difficulty in speaking and swollowing, etc. Cauliflower-like, nodular or helcoid masses can be found by nasopharyngoscope.

2. Qigong Treatment
1) Quiescent Sitting Health Cultivation Exercise
This exercise can be practised 3 to 4 times a day, 30 minutes each time. See Chapter Two for details.
2) Relaxed and Quiescent Recumbent Exercise

Practise 3 to 4 times a day, 30 minutes for each time. This exercise can be practised alternately with the Quiescent Sitting Health Cultivation Exercise.

3) Longevity Exercise

Practise 1 to 2 times a day, each time for 60 minutes. According to the conditions of the disease, the patient can select several parts of the exercise to practise. See Chapter Two for details.

4) Three Breathing Exercise

Stand and relax for 10 to 20 seconds with the mind concentrating on Shanzhong. Take 3 to 6 deep breaths through the nose only. Then begin walking. During the first two steps, inhale deeply 3 times. For example, take the first inhalation when the right foot steps forward, with the third inhalation coming when the left foot touches the ground. During the following two steps, make 3 exhalations. The heel should touch the ground first, then the tips of the toes. At the same time, shake the right arm, forming a figure 8. After the 3 inhalations and 3 exhalations, the shaking of the left arm should also be over. That is to say, inhale, inhale, and inhale again, and then exhale, exhale, and exhale again, with no breath holding and no discontinuation. Generally, the rate can be 20 to 25 times a minute, but slower for those with severe disease and weak health. The distance walked should be 1,000 to 3,000 meters, either going straight forward or walking in circles. In regulating the breath, the patient should listen to the sound of his or her own respiration. The same procedure should be followed when the left foot steps out first. Direct the *qi* with the mind, stimulating the circulation of the *zhen* (true) *qi*. This is called thoracic breathing. Sink the *qi* to Shanzhong, keeping it there the whole time. It is advisable to keep the heartbeat rate at below 100 times/min. In addition, this exercise can also be practised in the lying, sitting, standing or running posture.

3. Sample Case

Mr. Zhou, 38 years old, had been suffering from a stuffy nose due to cold for two years. The attacks of the disease were paroxysmal, and the patient often needed to breath with his mouth. He was diagnosed as having nasopharyngeal carcinoma after an examination in April 1979. After a chemotherapy for 5 months, his symptoms, such as deviation of the mouth, and difficulty in breathing still remained. Then, in March 1980, he began to receive treatment with traditional Chinese medicine supplemented with Qigong. Three months later, his condition had greatly improved. The deviation of the mouth was corrected and breathing could be done through the nose. The patient was normal with increased body weight, except for a mild congestion of the noseopharyngeal mucosa, and the mass had disappeared. He continued to practise Qigong for another 3 months, then stopping the drug treatment, although continuing the dietetic therapy. He returned to work in January 1981. In January 1982, he was found normal in the nasopharyngeal part. He is still practising Qigong in his spare time.

PULMONARY CARCINOMA

Pulmonary carcinoma, also called bronchopulmonary carcinoma, originates in the bronchial mucosa and is the most common malignant tumour of the lungs. This disease has a very high incidence, especially in male patients of over 40 years old.

1. Clinical Manifestations

Coughing, sputum with blood, hemoptysis, chest pain, shortness of breath, fever. In the late stage, there will be pathologic leanness, tiredness, low fever or cachexia.

2. Qigong Treatment

1) Quiescent Sitting Health Cultivation Exercise

Practise this exercise 3 to 4 times a day, 30 minutes for each time. See Chapter Two for details. For those with severe illness or weak constitutions, can practise Relaxed and Quiescent Recumbent Exercise instead.

2) Up-and-down Respiration-adjusting Exercise

Relax and stand with the legs a shoulder width apart. Keep calm, rid yourself of distracting thoughts and concentrate the mind on lower Dantian (Huiyin). Lift up both hands slowly from the front of the body, inhaling at the same time. When the hands reach the maximal point, turn them backwards. Then expire slowly while the hands are lowered along both sides of the body. Meanwhile, squat down, lowering the hands to the level of the lower Dantian, and at the same time sinking the *qi* to the lower Dantian. Then, with the ascending of the body, raise the hands along the front of the body. Move slowly, at a rate of 5 to 10 times a minute. Twenty-five times make one sequence. This exercise can be practised 3 times a day. Each time practise one sequence or several according to the health conditions.

3) Three Respiration Exercise

This exercise can be practised once or twice a day. See the previous section of nasopharyngeal carcinoma for details.

4) Anti-carcinoma Exercise I

Relax and stand with the hands overlapped at the middle Dantian (Qihai). For males, the left hand is put under the right hand, and for females, the right hand under the left one (Fig. 94-1). Close the mouth and inhale through the nose. Then exhale through the slightly opened mouth while relaxing the knees, hip and waist and slowly squatting down (Fig. 94-2). Then inhale again (note: begin to inhale before the last exhale is finished). After exhaling, stand up slowly. Repeat the movements three times (This is the so-called San Xi Xu). Then separate both hands, moving them towards the coastal regions with the back of the palms opposite to each other, until the separation is a little wider than the body (Fig. 94-3). Then turn over the hands so the palms face each other, and bring them slowly to the level of the middle Dantian. As the hands nearly touch each other (Fig. 94-4), turn them over again and do the second opening and closing. Repeat the movements three times (this is the so-called San Kai He). Then step forward the left foot and inhale, and step forward the right foot and exhale. Walk forward like this for 15 to 20 minutes, at a rate of 100 to 120 steps per minute. Perform San Xi Xu and San Kai He again before ending the exercise. This exercise can be practised 4 to 6 hours every day. However, it is harmful to those with ascites due to hepatic carcinoma, cirrhosis, anemia, urinaemia, heart disease, leukemia, pancreatitis and other gynecological diseases.

3. Sample Case

Mr. Yue, 42, had been in good health. In an examination, he was found to have a ball-like mass close to the right lower hilus of the lungs, diagnosed as pulmonary carcinoma. In an operation, the tumour, 7x8 cm in size, was found to have metastasized making an operation impossible. It was predicated that he could survive only 3 months. He began to practise Qigong two months after beginning radiotherapy, which improved his appetite and sleep. He gained weight and his blood picture gradually normalized. After practising for over one year, he began to enjoy good health again.

ESOPHAGUS CARCINOMA

Esophagus carcinoma is a common malignant tumour with high incidence in

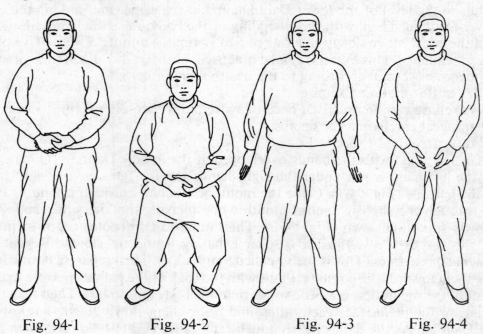

Fig. 94-1   Fig. 94-2   Fig. 94-3   Fig. 94-4

certain regions. It is very common in males of over 40 years old. The incidence in North China is higher than that in the south.

1. Clinical Manifestations

Continuous and progressive dysphagia, discomfort and pain in the chest, regurgitation, often complicated by celostomia, shortness of breath, dry coughing and hiccuping. In the late stage, there will be pathogenic weight loss, dehydration and anemia.

2. Qigong Treatment

1) Quiescent Sitting Health Cultivation Exercise

Practise 3 to 4 times a day, each time 30 minutes. See Chapter Two for details.

2) Relaxed and Quiescent Recumbent Exercise

This exercise can be practised in combination with the Quiescent Sitting Health Cultivation Exercise. Practise 3 to 4 times a day, each time 30 minutes. See Chapter Two for details.

3) Three Respiration Exercise

Practise once or twice daily. See the section of nasopharyngeal carcinoma.

4) Up-and-down Respiration-adjusting Exercise

Practise 3 times a day. See the section of pulmonary carcinoma.

5) Anti-carcinoma Exercise I

See the section of pulmonary carcinoma.

6) Exercise for Prevention and Treatment of Cancers

Relax and stand, performing San Xi Xu and San Kai He. Then step forward the left foot first and inhale, then the right foot and inhale again. On the third step, begin to exhale, but on the fourth step, when the right foot is stepping out, do not inhale or exhale. Four steps make up of one group. Walking 120 to 140 steps in one minute, the patient should walk 75 minutes for each practice. Practise 2 to 3 times each day. Attention should be paid that San Xi Xu and San Kai He should be performed again in ending each practice. This exercise can be practised with intervals for 4 to 6 hours every day. However it is harmful to those with cirrhosis, hepatic carcinoma, ascites, heart disease, urinaemia, severe anemia. These patients should avoid practising it.

3. Sample Case

Mr. Sun, 45 years old, suffered from dysphagia in June 1979. In September, the barium meal exam found the midsection of the esophagus to be blocked. The lesion was as long as 11.5 cm and the WBC was 11100. In an examination, it was found that the affected part had already ulcerated. The patient suffered difficulty in eating and drinking. He was diagnosed as having carcinoma in the middle section of the esophagus. The patient still had difficulty eating after radiotherapy of ten months and having traditional Chinese medicine of one and a half months. He began to practise Qigong in Feburary 1980. Some time later, the patient felt better in eating and sleeping. X-ray in June revealed that there was increased markings in both lungs, the heart was normal and the lungs were without metastases. In an examination in September showed that the lesion had disappeared. The barium meal could go through the esopagus freely and the lesion area had become normal. The patient continued to practise Qigong after returning to work.

STOMACH CARCINOMA

Stomach carcinoma is the most common malignant cancer in China, accounting for 50 percent of all the tumours in the digestive system, and 10 percent of all cases of malignant tumours. It is most common in middle-aged males.

1. Clinical Manifestations

Distension, discomfort and pain in the upper abdomen, anorexia, nausea and vomiting, hematemesis or hematochezia. In the late stage, there will be abdominal masses, ascites, lymphadenectasis and progressive emaciation, fever and cachexia.

2. Qigong Treatment

1) Three Respiration Exercise

Practise 1 or 2 times a day. See section of nasophayngeal carcinoma for details.

2) Anti-carcinoma Exercise II

Relax and stand to perform San Xi Xu and San Kai He. Step forward the left foot first and inhale and exhale. Then step forward the right foot and inhale and exhale. Two steps make one sequence. Walk 40 to 60 steps in one minute and walk continuously for 20 minutes. Before ending the exercise, perform San Xi Xu and San Kai He again. After that, relax and stand for a few seconds. This exercise can be practised 4 to 6 hours a day with intervals.

3) Up-and-down Respiration-adjusting Exercise

Practise three times a day. See the lung carcinom section for details.

4) Quiescent Sitting Health Cultivation Exercise or Relaxed and Quiescent Recumbent Exercise

This exercise can be practised 3 to 4 times a day, 30 minutes each time. See Chapter Two for details.

3. Sample Case

Mr. Zhi, 59 years old, had been suffering from gastritis for many years. The pain could be relieved when he took liquid food, but there was still nausea. He had received drug and injection treatment in the hospital, but no improvement. He was found to have a pale and yellowish complexion, was thin and weak with a weight of 43.5 kg and acratia. The X-ray barium meal and gastroscopic examination showed that there was canceration. An operation was suggested. The patient went home to practise Qigong every morning and evening for 3 hours. Two years later, he could eat bread and work. He could sleep and eat normally, with an increased body weight of 52 kg. Half a year later, a barium meal exmination showed no abnormalities in his digestive tract.

HEPATIC CARCINOMA

Hepatic carcinoma refers to malignant tumours in the liver cells and the bile duct. It is common in middle-aged male adults between 40 to 50 years old. Its onset is considered to be closely related to hepatitis B.

1. Clinical Manifestations

The main symptoms include progressive hepatomegaly, pain, jaundice, ascites, fever, acratia, pathogenic leanness, hemorrhages and positive *a*-fetoprotein.

2. Qigong Treatment

1) Quiescent Sitting Health Cultivation Exercise or Relaxed and Quiescent Recumbent Exercise

These two exercises can be practised alternately 3 to 4 times a day, 30 to 60 minutes each time, so as to increase the physique. See Chapter two for details.

2) Anti-carcinoma Exercise II

Practise 4 to 6 hours every day with intervals. Lessen the practice for severe cases and those who are weak. See the stomach carcinoma section.

3) Longevity Exercise

According to the conditions of the disease, select the 1st, 8th, 11th, 17th, 20st, 22nd or 25th posture for practise. Practise 4 to 6 times a day, each time 30 minutes. See Chapter Two for details.

4) Lying Respiration-adjusting Exercise

Lie on the back and naturally calm yourself. Overlap the hands on Laogong and put them under the head. One leg should be straightened and the other bent 60 to 90 degrees (Fig. 95). Slightly close the eyes, leaving some light to see upward. Concentrate the mind in the upper Dantian. Place the tongue on the upper palate, half close the mouth, keep the breathing deep, long, fine, even and stable, at a rate of 8 times a minute. Breathe like this for 20 to 50 times. Switch the position of the lower limbs 3 to 4 times during the practice. This exercise can be practised 4 to 6

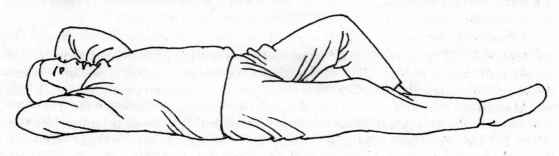

Fig. 95

times a day.

5) Three Respiration Exercise

This exercise can be practised according to the conditions of the disease.

BREAST CANCER

Breast cancer is a common malignant tumour in female patients, coming second after carcinoma of the uterus. In most cases, it occurs in females of 40 to 60 years old around the climacterium.

1. Clinical Manifestations

In the early stage, there are no symptoms and signs. Patients often find by accident small painless and solitary lumps in breasts. The lumps are hard in nature, with an unsmooth surface and unclear borderline. It is difficult to move them. Later the lumps will stick to the skin and there will be indentation in the skin, retracted or raised nipples, as well as hemolateral auxilliary lymphadenectasis.

2. Qigong Treatment

1) Quisecent Sitting Health Cultivation Exercise or Relaxed and Quiescent Recumbent Exercise

Practise these exercises 3 to 4 times a day, 30 minutes each time. See Chapter Two for details. These two exercises can be practised alternately. Those who lie in bed due to poor health can practise the lying exercise.

2) Three Respiration Exercise

Practice 1 time or 2 times a day. See the section of Nasopharyngeal carcinoma.

3) Up-and-down Respiration

Practise 3 times a day. See the section of pulmonary carcinoma.

4) Anti-carcinoma Exercise I and II

Practise one of the two exercises or do them alternately. See the sections of pulmonary carcinoma and stomach carcinoma.

5) Longevity Exercise

Select several sections according to the conditions of the disease. Practise 3 to 4 times a day, 30 minutes each time. See Chapter Two for details

3. Sample Case

Ms. Jiang, 42 years old, found by accident a small lump of about 1.5 cm in size on her right breast in May 1975. It was diagnosed as breast cancer. She underwent an immediate surgical operation. Two years later, she had an operation again due to metastasis of the carcinoma. This time, her ovaries were removed. After that, she was given radiotherapy and chemotherapy. From July 1977, she began to practise Qigong. Then the lesions in the left breast and sternal region resulting from the metastasis stopped developing, and such side effects of the radio and chemotherapy as poor appetite, poor sleep and acratia, all disappeared. She felt energetic and had a normal blood picture. So she went back to work.

CERVICAL CARCINOMA

Cervical carcinoma, a common gynecological malignant tumour, is most frequently found in married women between 35 to 55 years old.

1. Clinical Manifestations

There are often no obvious symptoms and signs at the early stage of the disease. Then there may be slightly-increased leukorrhea and a very small amount of contact hemorrhage or discontinuous postmenopausal bleeding. In the late stage, there will be increased vaginal secretion, hemorrhages, persistent pain in the lower abdomen, thighs and groin, etc. These are also complicated by frequent micturition, urgency of urination, urodynia and dysuria or dysporia and hematochezia.

2. Qigong Treatment

1) Quiescent Sitting Health Cultivation Exercise or Relaxed and Quiescent Recumbent Exercise

These exercises can be practised 3 to 4 times a day, each time for 30 minutes. According to the conditions of the disease, either or both of the exercises can be practised. See Chapter Two for details.

2) Anti-carcinoma Exercise I

Practise this exercise 4 to 6 hours every day with intervals. See the sections of carcinoma of the pulmonary and the esophagus.

3) Up-and-down Respiration-adjusting Exercise

Practise 3 times a day. See the section of pulmonary carcinoma.

4) Three Breathing Exercise

Practise 1 time or 2 times a day. See the section of nasopharyngeal carcinoma.

3. Sample Case

Ms. Wang, 42 years old, was diagnosed as having cervical carcinoma of the third stage in 1962. Surgical operation had become impossible for her, so she had to lie in bed at home. She suffered from weakness of the lower limbs, distension of the abdomen, loss of weight and poor appetite. No therapeutic effect was obtained after treatment with acupuncture, Chinese herbs and Western medicine. Her conditions, however, improved after 3 months of practice of Qigong, with increased body weight and decreased vaginal bleeding. Half a year later, there was no vagial bleeding. When she received reexamination in the hospital 9 months later, she was in perfect health.

MALIGNANT LYMPHOMA

Malignant lymphoma refers to a group of malignant tumours that involve the lymph nodes and lymph tissues.

1. Clinical Manifestations

Lymphadenectasis, hepatosplenomegaly, fever and cutaneous pruritus or various kind of skin rash, anemia, pathogenic leanness, etc.

2. Qigong Treatment

1) Quiescent Sitting Health Cultivation Exercise or Relaxed and Quiescent Recumbent Exercise

Practise 3 to 4 times a day, each time for over 30 minutes. Patient can practise one of the two exercises or practise them alternately according to the conditions of the disease. See Chapter Two for details.

2) Anti-carcinoma Exercise I or Exercise for Prevention and Treatment of Cancers

Practise these exercises 4 to 6 hours a day. See the section of nasopharyngeal carcinoma.

3) Three Respiration Exercise

Practise once or twice a day. See the section of nasopharyngeal carcinoma.

3. Sample Case

Mr. Cao, 65 years old, was diagnosed as having malignant lymphoma in September 1986. He received chemotherapy for 4 months, and the tumour was reduced in size. However, his state deteriorated due to emotional stress. There were six palpital lumps under his neck, armpits and in the groin which were as big as eggs with obvious hardness and pain. He began to practise Qigong in May 1987. Twenty days later, the pain became less severe and the lumps smaller. After he had practised Qigong for two months, all the six lumps had disappeared and the patient was in high spirits.

OSTEOSARCOMA

This is one of the malignant tumours of the bones. It is most common in young patients between 10 to 25 years old.

1. Clinical Manifestations

The main symptoms are persistent local pain, more severe at night, local palpable lumps with tenderness and peripheral myophagism, tension and shining of the skin surface on top of the lumps, complicated by anorexia, pathogenic leanness, low fever and anemia.

2. Qigong Treatment

1) Quiescent Sitting Health Cultivation Exercise or Relaxed and Quiescent

Recumbent Exercise

Practise 3 or 4 times a day, each time, for 30 minutes. Patient can practise one of the two exercises or do them alternately. See Chapter Two for details.

2) Longevity Exercise

Practise some sections of this exercise, 3 times a day, 30 minutes for each. See Chapter Two for details.

3) Anti-carcinoma Exercise I, or Exercise for Prevention and Treatment of Cancers

Practise 4 to 6 hours every day. See the section of pulmonary carcinoma and esophagus carcinoma.

4) The Five Animals Frolic

Practise 2 to 3 times a day, each time for 20 to 30 minutes. See Chapter Two for details.

3. Sample Case

Zhu, a young man of 17 years old, suffered from pain and functional disorder of the left arm. Gradually he lost motor ability to the extent that he had to be looked after by others. He was diagnosed as having osteolytic osteosarcoma. He underwent immunotherapy supported by diet therapy, as well as Qigong therapy. Six months later, the patient was found normal and returned to school. The 2-year follow-up survey found no deterioration. He insisted on practicing Qigong every morning and evening to consolidate the therapeutic effect.

Chapter Five
JINGLUO AND QIGONG POINT MASSAGE

THE DISTRIBUTION OF *JINGLUO* AND ITS FUNCTIONS

Jingluo is a general term for the meridians and collaterals in the human body. The meridians, which constitute the main trunks, run longitudinally and interiorly within the body; while the collaterals, which represent branches of the meridians, run transversely and superficially from the meridians. The *jingluo* are pathways in which the *qi* and blood of the human body are circulated. They pertain to the visceral organs and extend over the surface of the body, forming a network and linking the tissues and organs, such as the five visceral (*zang*) and six internal (*fu*) organs, four limbs and bones of the whole body, five sense organs and nine orifices, skin, muscles and tendons, into an organic whole.

1. The Twelve Regular Meridians

The twelve regular meridians include the three yin meridians of the hand (the lung, the pericardium and the heart), and the three yang meridians of the hand (the large intestine, the Sanjiao and the small intestine), the three yang meridians of the foot (the stomach, the gallbladder and the bladder), and three yin meridians of the foot (the spleen, the liver and the kidney). Since they belong to the twelve visceral organs and are the major trunks in the *jingluo* system, they are called *zheng jing* (the regular meridians). Their main functions are to connect the visceral organs and limbs and to transport *qi* and blood to nourish the whole body.

All those meridians belonging to the six visceral organs (heart, liver, spleen, lungs, kidneys and pericardium) are yin meridian, which will go along the medial sides of the four limbs, the chest and the abdomen after they leave the six visceral organs. Those distributed on the medial sides of the upper limbs are three yin meridians of the hand and those distributed on the medial sides of the lower limbs are the three yin meridians of the foot. All those meridians belonging to the six internal organs (gallbladder, stomach, small intestine, large intestine, Sanjiao and bladder) are yang meridians. After leaving the six internal organs, they will go along the lateral sides of the four limbs, the head, the face and the trunk. The ones that travel along the lateral sides of the upper limbs are the three yang meridians of the hand and the ones that travel along the lateral sides of the lower limbs are the three yang meridians of the foot. As to the distribution of the twelve regular

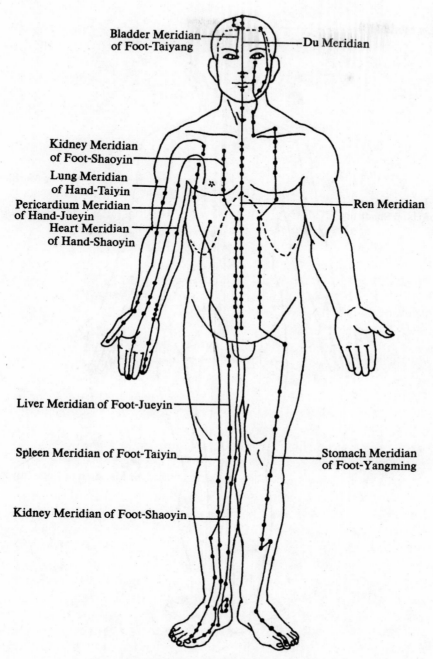

Fig. 96 Meridians (Front View)

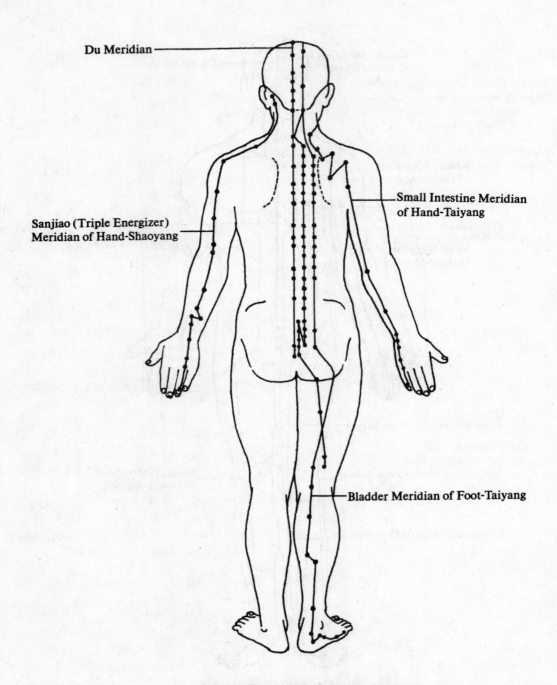

Fig. 97 Meridians (Back View)

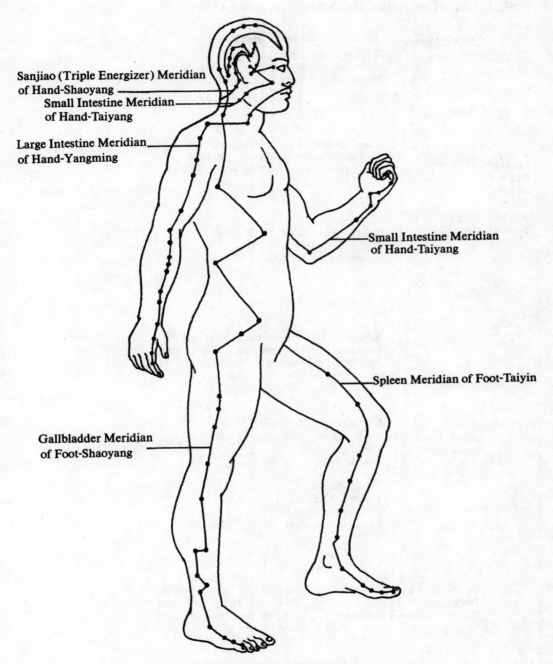

Sanjiao (Triple Energizer) Meridian
of Hand-Shaoyang
Small Intestine Meridian
of Hand-Taiyang

Large Intestine Meridian
of Hand-Yangming

Small Intestine Meridian
of Hand-Taiyang

Spleen Meridian of Foot-Taiyin

Gallbladder Meridian
of Foot-Shaoyang

Fig. 98 Meridians (Side View)

Table I. Classification of the Meridians and Collaterals

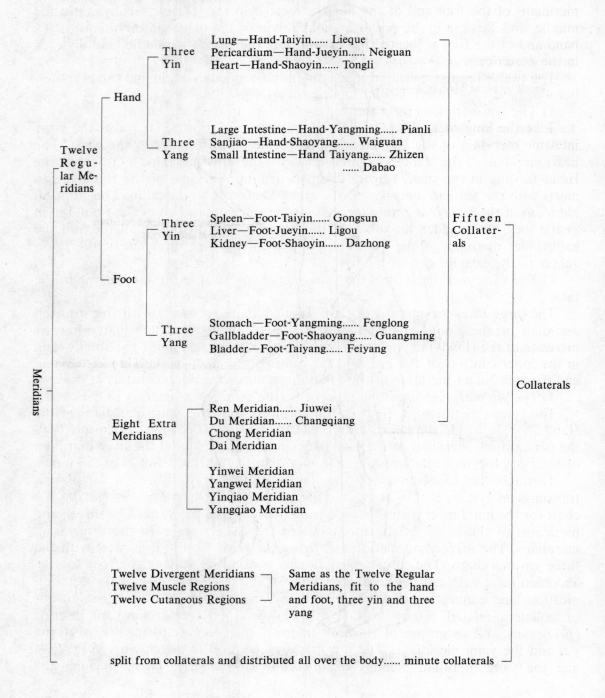

Three Yin
- Lung—Hand-Taiyin...... Lieque
- Pericardium—Hand-Jueyin...... Neiguan
- Heart—Hand-Shaoyin...... Tongli

Three Yang
- Large Intestine—Hand-Yangming...... Pianli
- Sanjiao—Hand-Shaoyang...... Waiguan
- Small Intestine—Hand Taiyang...... Zhizen
- ...... Dabao

Three Yin
- Spleen—Foot-Taiyin...... Gongsun
- Liver—Foot-Jueyin...... Ligou
- Kidney—Foot-Shaoyin...... Dazhong

Three Yang
- Stomach—Foot-Yangming...... Fenglong
- Gallbladder—Foot-Shaoyang...... Guangming
- Bladder—Foot-Taiyang...... Feiyang

Hand / Foot — Twelve Regular Meridians

Fifteen Collaterals

Eight Extra Meridians
- Ren Meridian...... Jiuwei
- Du Meridian...... Changqiang
- Chong Meridian
- Dai Meridian

- Yinwei Meridian
- Yangwei Meridian
- Yinqiao Meridian
- Yangqiao Meridian

Collaterals

Meridians

Twelve Divergent Meridians
Twelve Muscle Regions
Twelve Cutaneous Regions

Same as the Twelve Regular Meridians, fit to the hand and foot, three yin and three yang

split from collaterals and distributed all over the body...... minute collaterals meridians in the head, body and the four limbs, Yangming of the three yang meridians of the foot and of the hand is located in the interior, Shaoyang in the middle, and Taiyang in the posterior; and Taiyin of the three yin meridians of the hand and of the foot is located in the anterior, Jueyin in the middle, and Shaoyin in the posterior.

The twelve regular meridians have not only fixed localization and travel routes, but also have close interrelations among themselves.

1) The yin meridians meet the yang meridians in the four limbs.

Take the lung meridian of the Hand-Taiyin as an example. It meets the large intestine meridian of the Hand-Yangming in the posterior part of the wrist. The heart meridian of the Hand-Shaoyin meets with the small intestine meridian of the Hand-Taiyang in the small finger. The pericardium meridian of the Hand-Jueyin meets with the Sanjiao meridian of the Hand-Shaoyang in the palm. The stomach meridian of the Foot-Yangming meets with the spleen meridian of the Foot-Taiyin in the toes, the bladder meridian of the Foot-Shaoyin in the small toe and the gallbladder meridian of the Foot-Shaoyang with the liver meridian of the Foot-Jueyin in the exterior end of big toe.

2) The yang meridians meet the yang meridians bearing the same name in the face.

The large intestine meridian of the Hand-Yangming meets with the stomach meridian of the Foot-Yangming at the side of the nose. The small intestine meridian of the Hand-Taiyang meets with the bladder meridian of the Foot-Taiyang in the inner canthus of the eye, and the Sanjiao meridian of the Hand-Shaoyang and the gallbladder meridian of the Foot-Shaoyang in the outer canthus of the eye.

3) The yin meridians meet yin meridians (the three-yin meridians in the chest).

The spleen meridian of the Foot-Taiyin meets with the heart meridians of the Hand-Shaoyin inside the heart, kidney meridian of the Foot-Shaoyin meets with the pericardium meridian of the Hand-Jueyin in the chest, and the liver meridian of the Foot-Jueyin meets with the lung meridian of the Hand-Taiyin in the lung.

Through the connections of the Twelve Regular Meridians a circulating transmission system is thus formed. That is, the three yin meridians leaving the chest for the hand meet with the three yang meridians in the hand. The three yang meridians of the hand leaving the hand for the head meet with the three yang meridians. The three yang meridians leaving the head for the foot meet with the three yin meridians. The three yin meridians of the foot leaving the foot for the abdomen meet with the three yin meridians of the hand. Because of the communications and connection of the branch meridians and the collaterals, six groups of "collateral related" relations are formed between the visceral (*zang*) and interior (*fu*) organs, and six groups of "exterior-interior" relations are formed between the yin and the yang meridians. The yin meridian belongs to *zangluofu* (脏络腑), and the yang meridian belongs to *fuluozang* (腑络脏). Then, through the connection of the meridians bearing the same names of the hand and foot, a circulation system of the twelve regular meridians is formed. (See Table 2)

2. The Eight Extra Meridians

The eight extra meridians is the general term for the eight meridians, namely,

Table. 2 Connections of the Twelve Regular Meridians

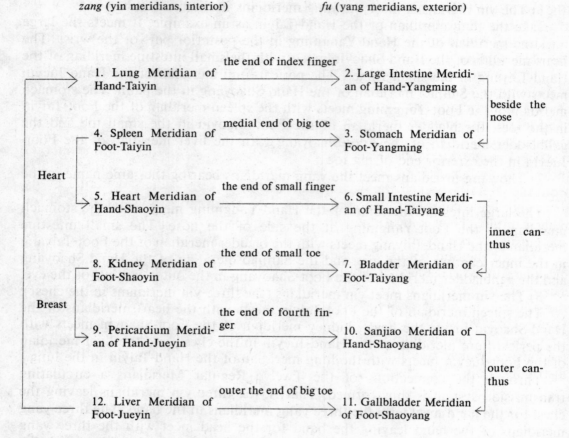

Du, Ren, Chong, Dai, Yinwei, Yangwei, Yinqiao and Yangqiao. Different from the twelve regular meridians, they neither pertain to the visceral organs nor communicate with the internal organs, neither pertain to the internal organs nor communicate with the visceral organs. They are not exteriorly-interiorly related. Their main functions are to control, store and regulate the circulation of qi and blood in the twelve regular meridians.

The Ren Meridian runs along the midline of the abdomen and the chest and goes upward to the chin, meeting all the yin meridians. Thus it is called "the sea of the yin meridians." It is responsible for all the yin meridians.

The Du Meridian runs along the midline of the back and ascends to the head and face, meeting all the yang meridians. Therefore it is called "the sea of the yang meridians." Its function is to govern the *qi* of all the yang meridians of the body.

The Chong Meridian runs parallel to the kidney meridian of Foot-Shaoyin up to the infra-orbital region, meeting all the twelve regular meridians. So it is called "the sea of the twelve meridians" or the "sea of blood." Its function is to store the *qi* and blood of the twelve regular meridians.

The Dai Meridian, which originates in the hypochondrium and goes around the waist binding up all the meridians.

The Yinwei Meridian is connected with the six yin meridians and meets at Ren Meridian; the Yangwei Meridian is connected with the six yang meridians, meeting at the Du Meridian. The two meridians regulate the flow of *qi* in the six yin and yang meridians, so as to maintain coordination and balance between the yin and yang meridians.

The Yinqiao Meridian starts from the medial aspect of the heel and merges into the meridian of Foot-Shaoyin to go upwards; the Yangqiao Meridian starts from the lateral aspect of the heel and merges into the meridian of Foot-Taiyang to ascend. Following their own courses, the two meridians meet each other at the inner canthus. They jointly regulate the motion of the lower limbs and opening and closing of the eyelids.

Most of the Shu points of the extra eight meridians are in the twelve regular meridians, only that the Ren, Du meridians have their own respective Shu points. Therefore, together with the twelve regular meridians, they are collectively called the fourteen meridians. As to the distribution of the fourteen meridians, see the figures from 96 to 101.

Generally, the meridians transport blood and *qi* to adjust yin and yang, nourish tendons and bones, and improve the joint function. A good master of the *jingluo* distribution can help practise Qigong and treat the diseases.

THE COMMONLY-USED QIGONG POINT MASSAGE

The Qigong point massage, a kind of Qigong massage on the acupoints of the human *jingluo*, is a substitution of the acupuncture therapy and herbal therapy. According to the theory that massage can relieve the pain and regulate the physiological functions of the body. This method can cure certain diseases without using needles and drugs, but using certain Qigong manipulation and selected acupoints.

1. The Commonly-used Points and Manipulations

The point massage can dredge the circulation of *qi* and blood, clear and activate the meridians and collaterals and strengthen the immunological and disease-resisting abilities of the body. It can also regulate *qi* and blood, balance yin and yang, enhance the body resistance to eliminate the pathogenetic factors, mobilize the potential energy of the body to achieve the goal of fighting against diseases and prolonging life. However manipulation and a correct selection of points according to the theory of traditional Chinese medicine is essential.

1) The commonly-used points and manipulations

The commonly-used points Baihui: on the midline of the head, approximately on the midpoint of the line connecting the apexes of the two ears.

Shangxing: 1 cun directly above the midpoint of the anterior hairline.

Yintang: midway between the medial ends of the two eyebrows.

Taiyang: in the depression about 1 cun posterior to the midpoint between the lateral end of the eyebrow and the outer canthus.

Yuyao: in the middle of the eyebrow directly above the pupil.

Zanzhu: in the depression proximal to the medial end of the eyebrow.

Sizhukong: in the depression at the lateral end of the eyebrow.

Jingming: 0.1 cun lateral and superior to the inner canthus.

Tongziliao: 0.5 cun lateral to the outer canthus.

Juliao: at the level of the lower border of ala nasi, on the lateral side of the nasolabial groove.

Chengqi: with the eyes looking straight forward, the point is directly below the pupil, between the eye ball and the infraorbital ridge.

Sibai: with the eyes looking straight forward, the point is nearly 1 cun under the pupil, in the depression at the infraorbital foramen.

Yingxiang: in the nasolabial groove, at the level of the midpoint of the lateral border of ala nasi.

Bitong: at the highest point of the nasolabial groove.

Jiache: one finger-breadth anterior and superior to the lower angle of the jaw at the prominence of the masseter muscle when the teeth are clenched.

Dicang: 0.4 cun lateral to the corner of the mouth.

Renzhong: a little above the midpoint of the philtrum, near the nostrils.

Chengjiang: in the depression in the centre of the mentolabial groove.

Tinggong: in the depression shown between the tragus and mandibular joint when the mouth is slightly opened.

Tinghui: anterior to the intertragic notch, at the posterior border of the condyloid process of the mandible.

Yifeng: posterior to the earlobe, in the depression between the mandible and mastoid process.

Fengchi: in the depression between the upper portion of m. sternocleidomastoideus and m. trapezius, on the same level with the inferior border of the mastoid process.

Fengfu: 1 cun directly above the midpoint of the posterior hairline, directly below the external occipital protuberance, in the depression between m. trapezius of both sides.

Jingzhong: 2 cun below the midpoint between Fengchi and Yiming, at the posterior of the m. sternocleidomastoideus.

Tianzhu: here it refers to the great occipital nerve at the back of the neck.

Touwei: 0.5 cun within the anterior hairline at the corner of the forehead.

Yangbai: on the forehead, 1 cun directly above the midpoint of the eyebrows.

Shangen: midpoint between the interior corner of the eyes.

Tiantu: in the centre of the suprasternal fossa.

Shanzhong: in the midway between the nipples.

Zhongwan: on the midline of the abdomen, 4 cun above the umbilicus.

Shuifen: on the midline of the abdomen, 1 cun above the umbilicus.

Tianshu: 2 cun lateral to the centre of the umbilicus (the point of the Stomach Meridian of Foot-Yangming).

Huangshu: 0.5 cun lateral to the umbilicus (the point of the Kidney Meridian of Foot-Shaoyin).

Qihai: on the midline of the abdomen, 1.5 cun below the umbilicus.

Guanyuan: on the midline of the abdomen, 3 cun below the umbilicus.

Zhongji: on the midline of the abdomen, 4 cun below the umbilicus.

Huiyin: between the anus and the scrotum in males and between the anus and the posterior labial commissure in females.

Dazhui: below the spinous process of the seventh cervical vertebra.

Mingmen: below the spinous process of the second lumbar vertebra.

Shenshu: 1.5 cun lateral to the third lumbar vertebra.

Changqiang: midway between the tip of the coccyx and the anus, locating the point in prone position.

Quchi: when the elbow is flexed 90 degrees, the point is in the depression at the lateral end of the transverse cubital crease, midway between Chize and the latera epicondyle of the humerus.

Shousanli: 2 cun below Quchi.

Hegu: the place in the coincident position of the transverse crease of the interphalangeal joint of the thumb with the margin of the web between the thumb and the index finger of the other hand. The point is at the highest spot of the muscle when the thumb and index finger are brought close together.

Waiguan: 2 cun above Yangchi between the radius and ulna.

Zhigou: 1 cun above Waiguan.

Yangchi: on the transverse crease of the dorsum of the wrist, in the depression lateral to the tendon of m. extensor digitorum communis.

Shaoshang: on the radial side of the thumb, 0.1 cun posterior to the corner of the nail.

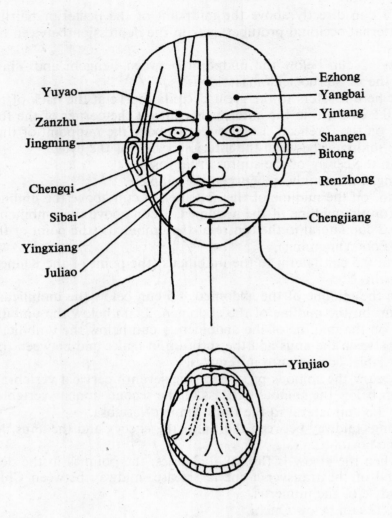

Fig. 99 Points on the Head, Face and Neck (Front View)

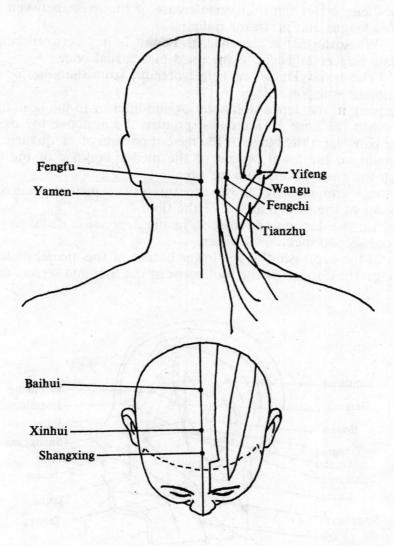

Fig. 100 Points on the Head, Face and Neck (Back View)

Neiguan: 2 cun above the transverse crease of the wrist, between the tendons of m. palmaris longus and m. flexor radialis.

Laogong: When the fist is clenched, the point is just between below the ring and the middle fingers, adjacent to the third metacarpal bone.

Zusanli: 3 cun below Dubi, one finger-breadth from the anterior crest of the tibia, in m. tibialis anterior.

Yanglingquan: in the depression anterior and interior to the head of the fibula.

Xuehai: when the knee is flexed, the point is 2 cun above the mediosuperior border of the patella, on the bulge of the medial portion of m. quadriceps femoris.

Yinlingquan: on the lower border of the medial condyle of the tibia, in the depression on the medial border of the tibia.

Sanyinjiao: 3 cun directly above the tip of the medial malleolus, on the posterior border of the medial aspect of the tibia.

Taichong: on the dorsum of the foot, in the depression distal to the junction of the first and second metatarsal bones.

Zhaohai: in the depression of the lower border of the medial malleolus.

Xingjian: on the dorsum of the foot between the first and second toe, proximal

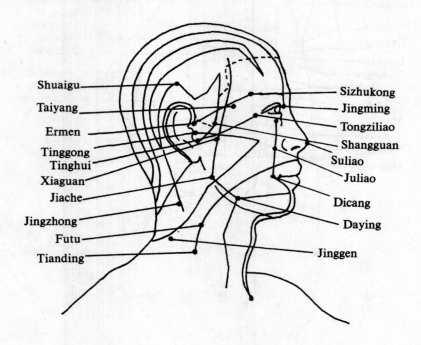

Fig. 101 Points on the Head, Face and Neck (Side View)

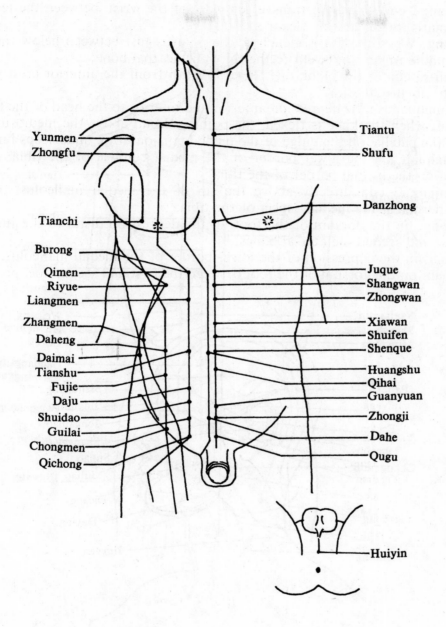

Fig. 102 Points on the Chest and Stomach

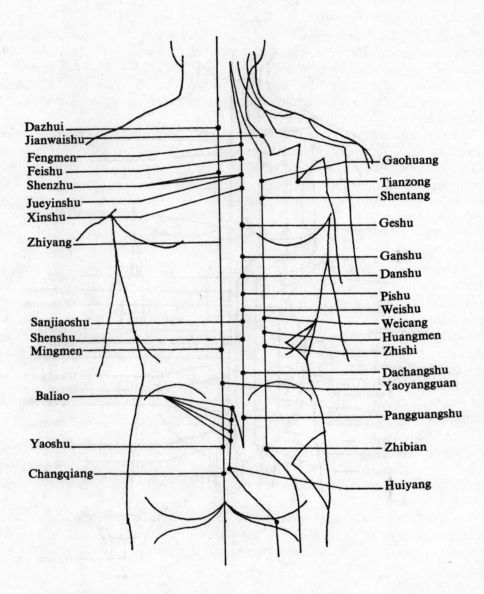

Fig. 103 Points on the Back and Waist

to the margin of the web.

Yongquan: on the sole, in the depression when the foot is in plantar flexion, approximately at the junction of the anterior third and posterior two-thirds of the sole.

Dantian: there are the upper Dantian (i.e. Shangen or Yintang), middle Dantian (Qihai), lower Dantian (Huiyin), interior Dantian (Shanzhong) and posterior Dantian (Mingmen).

Point Selection   The many points on the human body have their specific location. The accuracy of location of acupoints will affect the therapeutic effect. Great importance has always been attached to precise location of the points by medical practitioners in past ages. At present, commonly used are three methods of point selection: proportional measurement, anatomical landmarks and finger measurement.

2) The commonly-used manipulations of the point massage

a. Pressing

This method is divided into pressing with the thumb, pressing with the tips of the four fingers and pressing with the fist. This can be practised by putting the finger(s) on one or more points on the surface of the skin and applying proper pressure. This is applicable to all the points of the body. It has the function of clearing and activating the meridians and collaterals, and dissipating blood stasis and relieving the stagnation and removing the cold and stopping pain.

b. Digital point pressure

Pressing with strength on the point with the tip of the finger or olecranal part of the bent elbow. This is often used on the points of the waist, back and the four limbs. It has the functions of removing the cold and stopping pain.

c. Kneading

Knead the diseased part clockwise or counterclockwise with the palm, the base of the palm, the finger, the back of the hand or hypothenar. Its main functions are to remove local swelling and to eliminate the pathogenic wind and heat.

d. Clapping

Clap the diseased part with the palm or hypothenar. This can be performed by a single palm or both palms. It is applied to the shoulers, back, waist, chest, limbs, etc. It can help the circulation of *qi*, relax the muscles and relieve swelling and pain.

e. Rubbing

Rubbing the muscles of the diseased part up and down with the palm or the base of the palm with no intermission. It is often used on the waist, the buttocks and the four limbs. To prevent injury, some talcum powder can be used. This method has the function of soothing the liver, calming the liver to stop the wind and regulating *qi* and blood.

f. Pushing

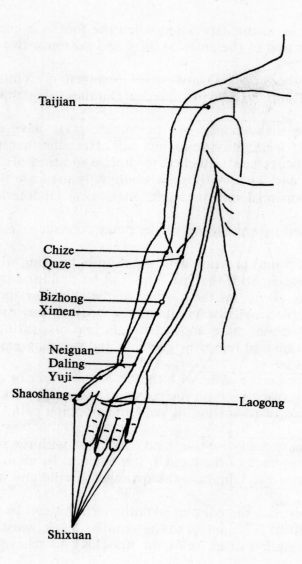

Fig. 104 Points on the Upper Limbs

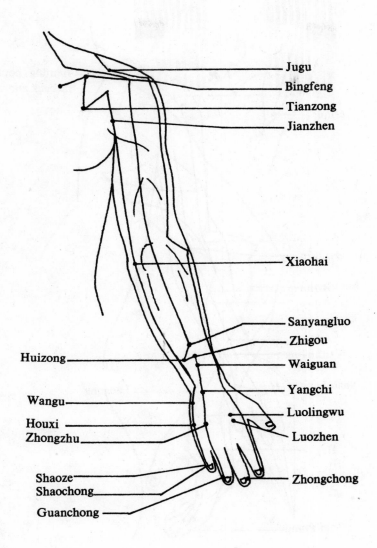

Fig. 105 Points on the Upper Limbs

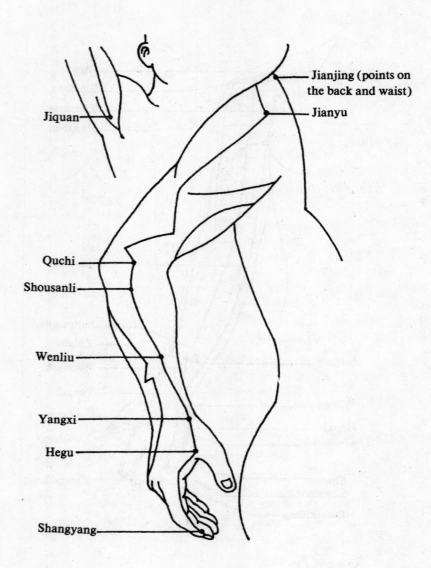

Fig. 106 Points on the Upper Limbs

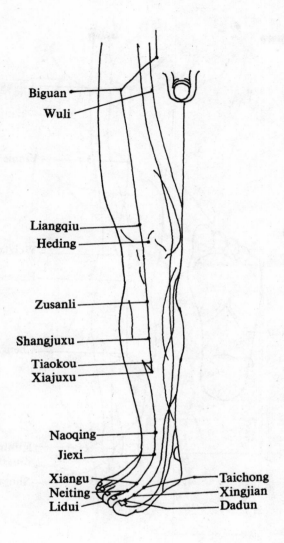

Biguan
Wuli
Liangqiu
Heding
Zusanli
Shangjuxu
Tiaokou
Xiajuxu
Naoqing
Jiexi
Xiangu
Neiting
Lidui
Taichong
Xingjian
Dadun

Fig. 107 Points on the Lower Limbs

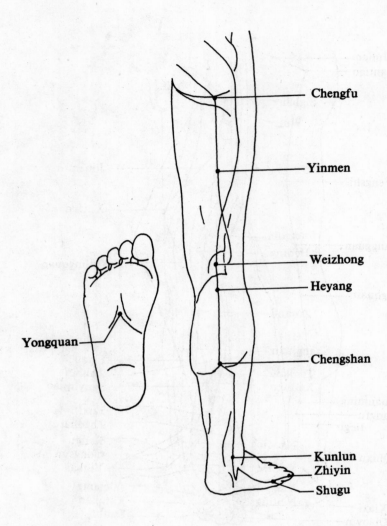

Fig. 108 Points on the Lower Limbs

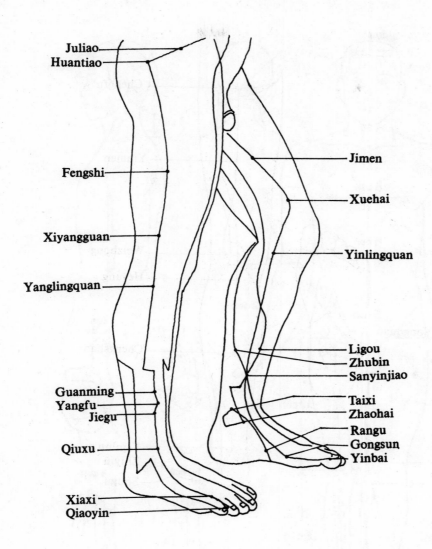

Juliao
Huantiao
Fengshi
Xiyangguan
Yanglingquan
Guanming
Yangfu
Jiegu
Qiuxu
Xiaxi
Qiaoyin

Jimen
Xuehai
Yinlingquan
Ligou
Zhubin
Sanyinjiao
Taixi
Zhaohai
Rangu
Gongsun
Yinbai

Fig. 109 Points on the Lower Limbs

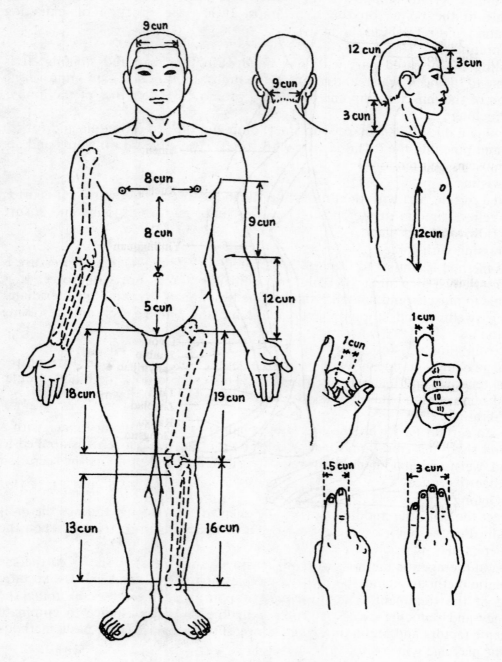

Fig. 110

Pushing a certain point with the thumb and other fingers with force. It is applicable to the points on the four limbs. It has the function of inducting resuscitation and refreshing the mind.

g. Rotating

Holding the diseased part with one hand or both hands and shaking. It is applicable to the neck, waist, and joints of the limbs. Its function is to improve the condition of the muscles, skin and joints and promote the activities of the limbs.

h. Pinching

Forming a duck-billed shape with the thumb and the index, middle and fourth fingers and pinching the diseased part with force. Then pinch downwards and act on the muscles and tendons.

i. Twisting

Hold a certain part with the thumb and the index finger and twist it . It is often used to relieve rigidity in the ends of the four limbs and small joints and ensure natural flow of *qi* and blood.

j. Pressing with force

This method is similar to the pressing of item a, only the degree of pressure is different. Item a is a light pressing and item i is a pressure with force. It is applicable to muscles and tendons, and has the function of dredging the meridians, subduing swelling and stopping pain and removing blood stasis and resolving stagnation.

k. Strumming

As if playing a guitar, move the thumb or other four fingers to and fro on the muscles, tendons, and ligaments of the body. This can promote the blood circulation and remove blood stasis, break up adhesion and relieve spasms.

l. Vibrating

Press a certain part with the overlapped palms or the tip of the finger with a quick and rhythmic vibration, forming a local vibrating feeling. This is applied to the head, waist and abdomen. It can regulate the nerves and promote the secretion of the digestive juices.

m. Qigong

Direct the *qi* to the middle Dantian and then to Neiluogong. Release the *qi* at this point. Put the point on the diseased part or the point to be treated. Then the goal of treatment is reached.

Several therapeutic methods of point massage　According to the TCM theory, therapeutic methods include both the principles of the treatment and the specific method of the treatment. The principles of point massage are reinforcing the deficiency and reducing excess, strengthening the body's resistance to eliminate pathogenic factors and regulating *ying* and *wei*. Following are some basic methods for point massage which should be mastered:

a. The warming method

This method of warming the yang and clearing pathogenic cold is used to treat the disease due to cold of the deficiency type. The disease is located mainly in the interior or both the interior and the exterior. Such manipulations as Qigong, pressing, and kneading can be practised on some fixed points, such as Qihai, Guanyuan, Shenshu and Baliao. It is required that the movement should be soft and swift so that heat can be produced. When the heat goes deep into the skin, muscles or visceral and internal organs, it can warm both the exterior and interior and remove the pathogenic cold.

b. The heat-clearing method

This method is often used to clear away pathogenic heat. It is effective in the case of excessive pathogenic heat or pathogenic heat in the interior. Its function is to clear away pathogenic heat, regulate yin and safeguard the body fluid and resolve thirst. As the symptoms of the diseases with a heat nature are very complicated and the pathogenic heat is divided into the heat in Qifen, Xuefen and Yingfen, a careful investigation of the disease before the treatment is important. For coma with a high fever, a quick and strong clearing is essential, otherwise the disease will become critical. For those with deficiency syndrome, clearing plus strengthening the body's resistance should be conducted so as to remove the pathogenic factors. The manipulation should be practised according to the conditions of the disease and the state of the pathogenic heat. Point massage on Renzhong and Shixuan to cure heatstroke can serve as an example.

c. The reinforcing method

This is a method to reinforce impaired *qi* and blood, yin and yang or visceral and internal organs, so as to support the body's resistance, remove the pathogenic factors, regulate yin and yang and supplement *qi* and blood. It is often used in cases of insufficiency of *qi* and blood, deficiency of the spleen and stomach and night sweating and emission and so on. The points selected include Zhongwan, Tianshu, Qihai, Guanyuan, Pishu and Weishu. The manipulations used are pushing and pressing. From the point of view of transmission via meridians, manipulations moving along the direction of the transmission is reinforcement. As to the degree of the stimulation, light stimulation is reinforcement. As for the direction of the blood flow, manipulation with a concentric nature is reinforcement, and clockwise rotation of the manipulation is reinforcement.

d. The reducing method

This is a method of reducing excess found in such cases as excessive heat in the Sanjiao, vexation and thirst, indigestion, difficulty in urination and defecation. Pushing and kneading are often used first on Shenque and Tianzhu and then on Changqiang. Going against the direction of the meridian transmission is reducing; strong stimulation is reducing; centrifugal manipulation is reducing, and counterclockwise manipulation is reducing.

e. The dredging method

This method is used to dredge the blockages. It can regulate *ying* and *wei*, dredge the meridians, remove the pathogenic factors and induce the production of body fluid. It can solve the problems of generalized swelling, numbness of the muscles and blocked meridians. A manipulation with both strength and gentleness can be used in the treatment. The commonly used methods are pushing and pressing.

f. The mediation method

This method is often used to treat the half exterior and half interior syndromes. The manipulations used are pushing, rubbing and Qigong. These should be done according to the condition of the disease. Its function is to mediate the vital essence of the body.

g. The diaphoretic method

This method is often used to treat diseases with diaphoretics, mainly for the exterior syndromes of the wind-cold type or the wind-heat type. For the cold due to wind-cold, the manipulation should change from lightness to heaviness. When sweating occurs, the purpose of eliminating pathogenic wind and cold is reached. For the cold due to wind-heat, the manipulation should be light and soft and overly heavy stimulation should be avoided. Those points that have the functions of inducing warmness and hotness, eliminating cold and wind, such as Fengchi, Fengfu, Quchi, Hegu, Dazhui and Weizhong, should be selected. The main manipulations used are pushing and pressing.

h. Resolving and dispersing

These two methods of point massage have very satisfactory results. Their main functions are dispersing and resolving. For such visible lesions as tumours, dispersing is used, and for such invisible lesions as pathogenic wind in the abdomen, resolving is used. Mainly pushing, rubbing, kneading and clapping are used to disperse the tumours, sputum stagnation and stagnancy of the turbid *qi*.

2. The Manipulations of Qigong Point Massage

1) Massaging the points in the head

a. Yintang

Take a sitting position. When the mind is calmed, the "three inhalation and exhalation" and "three times opening and closing" are performed (see Chapter Four). In both cases, exhalation should be done first. Then press the middle finger of the left hand on Yintang and put the middle finger of the right hand on the nail of the left middle finger. Turn the finger leftward nine times and then rightward nine times. Then perform point respiration three times. (Fig.111)

b. Baihui and Shuaigu

Put both palms on the head with the midline between the palm and the wrist on the tips of the ears and the middle fingers overlapped. Massage both points simultaneously with the palms and tips of the middle fingers, nine times forwards and nine times backwards. Then perform three times on point respirations. (Fig. 112)

c. Fengfu

Turn the middle finger on the Fengfu points leftward and rightward nine times respectively and then perform point respiration. Then massage the vagus nerve at the back of the ears with the four fingers moving down to the cheeks. Lower the hands to the Dantian. (Figs. 113-1, 2)

d. Yangbai and Tianzhu

Massage the Yangbai points. Turn inward nine times and outward nine times, then perform point respiration. Then move the hands to the head, massaging the scalp and then pinching Tianzhu. Pinch six times and massage six times (Figs. 114-1, 2). Then massage the back of the neck and then the front of the neck. Then lower the hands to the Dantian.

e. Touwei and Fengchi

Press Touwei with the middle fingers turning inward and outward nine times respectively. Then perform point respiration. Then press Fengchi, turning inward and outward nine times respectively, and perform point respiration again. Then lower the hands to the Dantian along the anterior part of the cheeks. (Figs. 115-1, 2)

f. Taiyang

Lift both hands to the level of the brow and rub from the brow to Taiyang. Turn anterior and posterior nine times respectively, and then perform point respiration. After the massage, clap the face to the cheeks with the fingers and then lower the hands to Dantian.

g. Sizhukong

Lift both hands to the level of the brow and rub from the brow to Sizhukong. Turn anterior and posterior nine times respectively, then perform point respiration. Clap the face to the cheeks with the four fingers of each hand and then lower

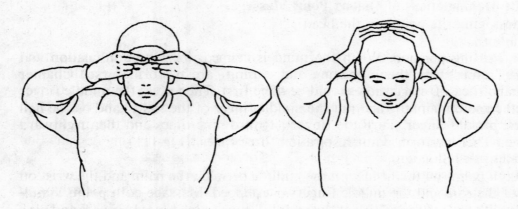

Fig. 111   Fig. 112

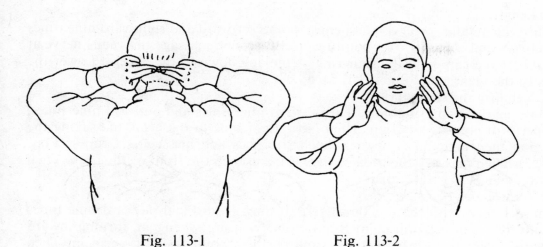

Fig. 113-1   Fig. 113-2

the hands to Dantian.

h. Points on the ears

Lift the hands to Yintang and massage under the brow to the anterior part of the ears. Press Xiaguan with the middle finger and Tinggong with the index finger, and then turn simultaneously forward and backward nine times. Then perform point respiration and lower the hands to Dantian. (Fig.116)

i. Points around the eyes

Press the small finger on Jingming and turn outward and inward nine times respectively. Perform point respiration. Then rub the orbit three times. (Fig. 117)

j. Points on the nose

Rub the sides of the nose with both middle fingers from up to down six times and then massage Yingxiang outward and inward nine times respectively. Perform point respiration. Then slip the fingers along the corners of the mouth to Chengjiang.

k. Chengjiang

Press the index fingers on Chengjiang, turning them inward and outward for nine times respectively, then perform point respiration (Fig.118). Lower the hands to Dantian. Then lift the hands to the hairline and rub the scalp from the anterior part to the posterior part, from the neck along the vagus nerve to the chin. Then lower the hands to Dantian. Repeat the movement nine times. At the ninth time when the hands lower to Dantian, perform "three times opening and closing and three times inhalation and exhalation." Then include the exercise.

This exercise requires that the ten fingers of the hands should be used to massage the points in the head and neck, so that such effects as clearing and activating the meridians and collaterals, promoting *qi* and blood circulation on the head, nourishment of blood and strengthening the functions of the brain, tonifying

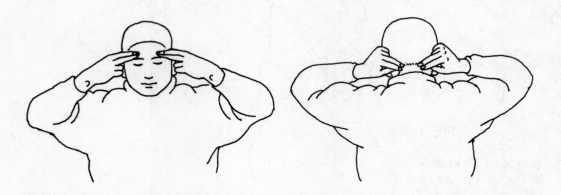

Fig. 114-1   Fig. 114-2

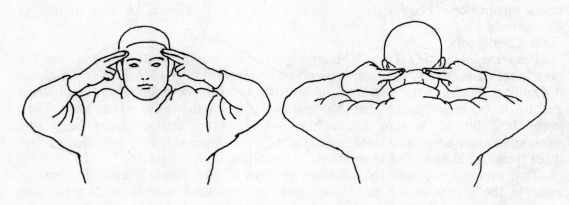

Fig. 115-1   Fig. 115-2

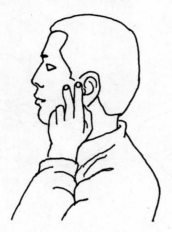

Fig. 116

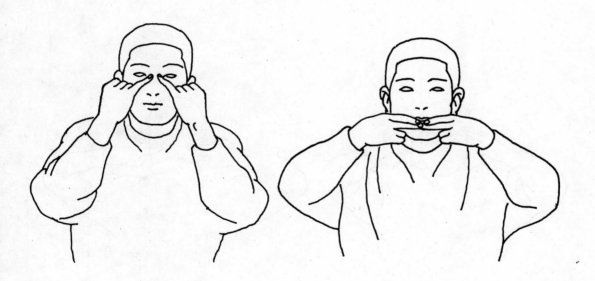

Fig. 117   Fig. 118

the heart and calming the mind as well as checking exuberant yang to easing mental strain can be achieved. This exercise can be used to treat dizziness, headaches, insomnia, tinnitus, nose diseases, eye diseases as well as apoplexy, facial paralysis, hemiplegia, disorders of stomach, proctoptosis and hematopathy.

2) Expectant Point Massage

See Chapter Three for details.

Chapter Six
QIGONG MASSAGE FOR NATURAL BEAUTY

Qigong, mainly through calisthenics or massage, can be used to improve the internal factors of the body, adjust the functions of the nervous system, regulate the balance of the body fluid and promote the metabolism. Different from the ordinary cosmetic methods, it not only beautifies the human figure and skin, but also helps regulate the functions of the internal organs and to promote health.

USING QIGONG TO MAKE THE FACE MORE BEAUTIFUL

Facial massage can promote the blood circulation and lipa secretion, eliminate wrinkles and get rid of fatigue. There are various ways of massage. Generally an effective massage should include the following three factors. First, the massage should be directed against the expressional wrinkle lines. In this way it can prevent those transverse wrinkles on the forehead, nose bridge, neck and so on. Second, it should promote blood circulation. For the radial wrinkles around the mouth and eyes, a circular massage is advisable. And third, it should press the nerve plexus. The pressure can relax the nerves and eliminate tiredness.

1. Getting Rid of Wrinkles at the Corners of the Eyes

The appearance of wrinkles at the corners of the eyes is a symbol of aging. Many people, especially women, are afraid of the appearance of this kind of wrinkles. However, it is simple to get rid of them, and usually a massage therapy of one week can achieve satisfactory results.

1) Put both index fingers on the Jingming points and press forcefully 5 times in 5 seconds.

2) Press Chengqi vertically with the index finger 5 times in 5 seconds.

3) Perform point-stimulation at 0.2 to 0.3 cun from the outer canthus 5 times in 5 seconds.

4) Press the points on the bladder meridian (see Chapter Five).

5) Press the points on the stomach meridian.

6) Press the points on the gallbladder meridian.

2. Getting Rid of Tiredness of the Eyes

A pair of glowing eyes plays an important role in cosmetology. Overuse of the eyes result in tiredness of the eyes and the loss of their beauty. Qigong massage can be used to get rid of the tiredness of the eyes.

1) Stimulate Jingming 5 times with both middle fingers and direct the force of the fingers toward the nose. Each time for 5 minutes. Then repeat.

2) Press Chengqi 5 times with both middle fingers.

3) Press Tongziliao 5 times with both middle fingers.

4) Lightly press the eyes with the index and the middle fingers while using the four fingers to press and pull the eyelids outwards 5 times. Attention should be paid that middle finger does not exert any force on the eyes. (Fig.119)

5) Make strong stimulation on Hegu with both thumbs 5 times.

6) Open the eyes and turn the eyeballs 5 rounds clockwise and then 5 rounds counterclockwise.

3. Making Yourself "Shining and Bright"

Qigong massage can make one "shining and bright," since massage can promote blood circulation, dilate the capillaries in the skin and enhance the metabolism. In addition, it can also regulate the central nervous system and relieve muscular spasms and physical tiredness.

1) First rub the face with both hands from the lower jaw to the top of the head, and then from the top of the head to the back of the ears, and back to the lower

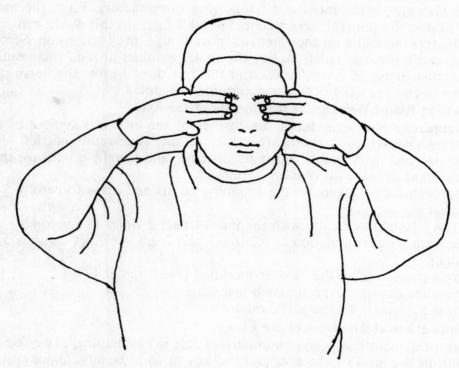

Fig. 119

jaw. Repeat more than ten times.

2) Knead the two small pits between the corners of the eyes and the nose bridge with the middle fingers for two minutes. Then knead Sibai slowly in circles for two minutes.

3) Bend the thumb and hold the thumb tips with the other four fingers. Rub the upper eyelids with the backs of the thumbs a dozen times. Then pull the eyelids slightly outwards three to five times.

4) Pinch Hegu until there is a sore and distended sensation. First pinch the left Hegu with the right hand for one minute and then pinch the right Hegu with the left hand for one minute.

5) Rub the palms until there is a sensation of warmth, then rub the face quickly 20 to 30 times.

6) Rub Shenshu repeatly and with force.

4. Preventing and Eliminating Freckles

Freckle are black or brown pigmentations. They commonly appear in young people around puberty or in pregnant women.

1) Press the lateral side of the heels along the bladder meridian, from the higher level to the lower level, 5 times.

2) Press Shugu posterior to the head of the fifth metatarsal bone for one minute. Repeat 5 times.

3) Massage the lumbodosal line from the top to the bottom 5 times. Then, with the spinal column as the middle line, press outwards to both sides with the palms more than ten times.

4) For freckles occurring in puberty, brush from the medial part of the thigh to the heel of both legs with a brush 10 times.

5. Eliminating Neoplasms on the Check

The face looks very unpleasant if there are neoplasms on it. The best way to remove these is by massage. The specific method is to push up from the lower jaw in the direction of the ears, hold the neoplasm with the fingers, and then put it down. Repeat the movements.

6. Facial Exercises

Facial calisthenics can make the muscles of the face and neck firm and soft. The calisthenics can be divided into two parts: simple facial movement and complicated movement.

1) Simple facial movement:

a. Slightly open the mouth and fill it with air. Then blow slightly. Inhale and blow like this again and again.

b. Move the lower jaw, as if chewing gum.

c. Open the mouth wide and close it tightly, again and again.

Each time the above movements can be performed for 10 minutes. Do them twice a day, once in the morning and once in the evening.

2) Complicated facial movement:

a. Lift the head slowly, turn it to the right and downwards and then left and downwards.

b. Raise the head backward as far as possible, and then restore to the original position. Repeat this several times.

c. Lift the muscles of both cheeks upwards with the thumbs and the index fingers.

d. Shake the head first to the right shoulder and then to the left one. Put the hands on the shoulders so that the shoulder will not move with the head.

Each of the above movements should be practised more than 20 times a day.

USING QIGONG TO MAKE THE NECK MORE BEAUTIFUL

The neck can easily show one's age. This is because the skin of the neck is loose and wrinkles may appear there earlier than on the face. For the sake of beauty, both facial and neck cosmesis are important, especially for females.

1. Raise the head backward as far as possible. Cover the upper lip with the lower lip. Then lower the head slowly until the lower jaw touches the chest. Repeat 4 to 6 times.

2. Turn the head slowly right and then left 4 to 6 times. Then do the same swiftly 8 to 10 times.

3. Turn the head slowly and then raise it. Repeat the movement 4 times for each side.

4. Turn the head to touch the shoulder, 4 to 6 times for each side. Do not lift the shoulders.

5. Tilt the head first to the right then to the left, with the ear touching the shoulder. Practise 4 to 6 times for each side.

6. Turn the head clockwise, then counterclockwise, 6 to 10 times for each direction.

7. Raise the lower jaw and restore the position, then lower the jaw until it reaches the chest. Repeat this movement 4 to 6 times.

8. Interlace the fingers and put them at the back of the head. First lower the head, and then raise the head backwards swiftly and forcefully, 4 to 6 times.

9. Place both elbows on the table, supporting the lower jaw with the overlapped hands. Push up the lower jaw and then lower the head. Repeat 4 to 6 times.

After the above-mentioned exercises are practised 10 to 12 days, double the times of the practice. Then increase the practice to 20 to 25 times a day.

EXERCISES FOR FEMALE BEAUTY

The chest, abdomen and buttocks are the most important parts of a woman's beauty. Practising these exercises can prolong a beautiful figure.

1. Exercises for Chest

Exercises for chest can promote the healthy development of the breasts, make them fuller and give them more elasticity. It can also regulate the postition of the breasts.

1) Stand straight. First straighten the chest and then retract the chest for 8 times.

2) Stand straight. Pull in the chest with lowering head and protruding shoulders. Then extend the chest as much as possible. Repeat 8 times.

3) Do exercise 1) again but the practice should be swifter and more forceful. Also repeat 8 times.

4) Stand straight. Expand the chest with bent arms and then straightened arms. Repeat 8 times.

5) Stand straight. First lower the head and pull in the chest with the arms crossing in front of the body. Raise the arms, chest and the head and sway to one side. Then raise up the arms while stretching out the chest and sway them. Repeat 8 times. Exhale when contracting the chest and inhale when lifting the chest.

6) Kneel down with the buttocks resting on the shanks, stretch the arms forward and expand the chest. Slip the body forward with the clavicle and chest touching the ground until in a prone position. Stretch the arms forward again, then bend the arms at the albows and raise the body with the support of the arms, slowly moving the body backward. Expand the chest again while raising the head, lowering the waist and lifting the buttocks. Throw out the chest as much as possible. Then return to the kneeling position (Figs. 120-1, 2, 3). Repeat 3 times.

2. Exercises for Abdomen

1) The lateral abdomen. Lie on the back. Do a sit-up and hold the right knee with the hands. Lie down again. Then do a sit-up again and hold the left knee this time. Repeat 8 times.

2) The lower abdomen. Lie on the back and straighten the toes. First retract the abdomen and raise the legs. Control the legs with the abdominal muscles, putting them down slowly. Don't bend the knees. Repeat 8 times.

3) The upper abdomen. Lie on the back. Put the arms at the sides of the body. First contract the abdomen with force, do a sit-up and return to the original position. When lie down again, make the spinal column touch the ground slowly from the lower part to the upper part. Repeat 8 times.

4) The whole abdomen. Put the arms on the sides of the body and straighten the toes. Do a sit-up, then hold the knees with both hands. Return to the original

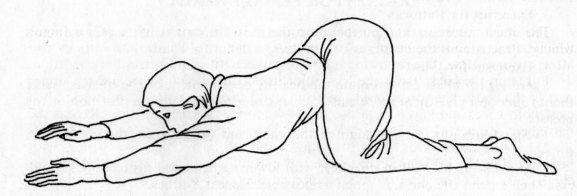

Fig. 120-1

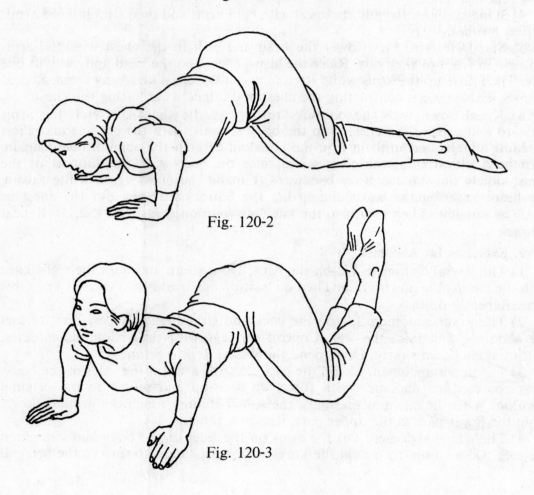

Fig. 120-2

Fig. 120-3

position. Repeat 8 times.

3. Exercises for Buttocks

Too much accumulation of subcutaneous fat in the buttocks is a major factor which detracts from the beauty of the body. On the other hand, flat buttocks also affects your outline. The following exercises can benefit women in either condition.

1) Lie on the back. Bend the legs 90 degrees. Lift the buttocks and the upper part of the body. The force should be from the contracted buttocks muscles. Then close both knees and lower the buttocks slowly to the original position. Repeat the movement 4 times. (Fig.121)

2) Lie face downwards . Rest the head on the bent arms and raise the legs with bent feet (Fig.122-1). Then separate the legs and raise the legs again with bent feet (Fig.122-2). Lift the legs with straightened feet alternately twice (Fig.122-3). Repeat this movement 4 times. It is required that the buttocks muscles should exert strength in the whole process and that the knee joints should be straight.

3) Support the body with the hands and knees with the upper part of the body resting slightly backward. Kick the legs alternately to the back and upwards (Fig.123). Repeat 4 times. During kicking, move the body a little bit forward, throw out the chest and contract the buttocks muscles on the movement side, so that the buttocks muscles can be raised.

SLIMMING FOR FEMALES

Most females prefer being slim. The following *jingluo* stimulation method can help them achieve this in three months.

Stimulate the seven meridians which are related to beauty with a towel or a brush during bathing every day.

1. Stimulate the foot-liver and -kidney meridians

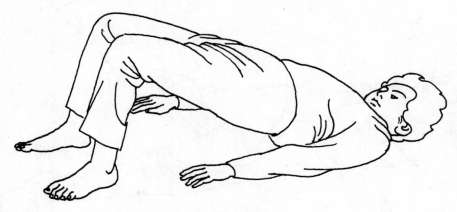

Fig. 121

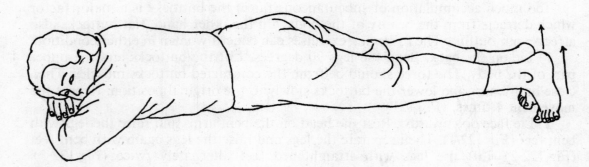

Fig. 122-1

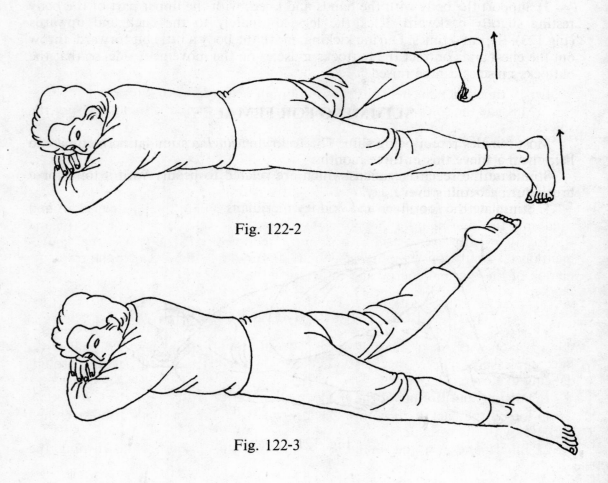

Fig. 122-2

Fig. 122-3

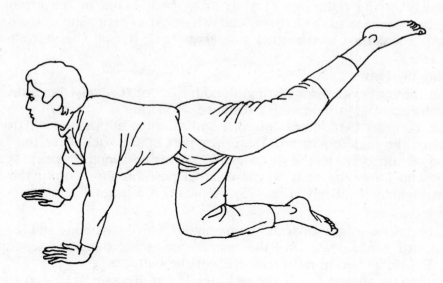

Fig. 123

Do 10 times of light helicoid stimulation all over the medial foot.

2. Massage the soles with the hand or a brush, especially the middle part of the sole.

3. Rub with force along the stomach meridian of the foot from the upper to the lower, 5 times.

4. Rub with force the bladder meridian of the foot from the upper to the lower to produce helicoid stimulation.

5. Brush with force along the large-intestine meridian, Sanjiao meridian and small-intestine meridian 5 times from the shoulder down to the tips of the fingers.

Together with exercises of the chest, abdomen and buttocks, the above-mentioned stimulations can intensify the body functions to normalize the transformation of the thermal energy and to beautify the body.

BODY-SHAPING EXERCISES

A person with fat or flaccid muscles, from any point of view, will make you look unpleasant. These exercises will help you keep a beautiful figure through dancing-like exercises.

1. Twisting and Rolling of the Body

1) Lie on the back with both knees bent to the chest and both arms stretched out level with the shoulders.

2) Inhale and rest the shoulders tightly on the ground while turning the

buttocks slowly to the right side. Try to bring both knees to the ground and meanwhile turn the head to the left side and exhale. After returning to the original position, inhale and turn to the other side (Fig. 124). Repeat this movement 25 times.

2. Raising the Pelvis

1) Lie on the back with arms resting on both sides of the body. Bend the knees and put the feet on the ground with a distance of 30 cm.

2) Inhale, contract the buttocks muscles and raise the buttocks slowly to make the lower part, the middle part and the upper part of the back leave the ground until the body is supported by the shoulders. Keep this position for several seconds. Then exhale and lower the body to the original position slowly until the spinal colomn is straightened entirely (Fig. 125). Repeat this 5 times.

3. Lifting the Legs

1) Lie face downwards, with arms resting on the sides of the body and the palms facing downward. Make one side of the cheeks touch the ground and separate the legs 15 cm. Exhale and contract the muscles of the buttocks.

2) Straighten the toes and raise the right leg 15 cm. Remain in this position for 1 second, and then put the leg down slowly. The pelvis should be kept against the ground. After this movement is repeated 50 times, do it again for another 50 times with the left leg. (Fig. 126)

4. Swinging and Kicking the Legs

1) Lie face downwards with bent arms and out-stretched hands with a shoulder width apart. Put the palms and pelvis tightly against the ground and raise both legs simultaneously for 15 cm.

2) Stablize the breathing and contract the muscles of the buttocks. Move the legs up and down as in free style swimming. Do this 50 to 100 times for each leg. (Fig.127)

5. Kicking in a Kneeling Position

1) Support the body with the hands shoulder width apart and knees at a distance of 20 to 30 cm. Straighten the right leg and raise it 30 cm from the ground.

2) Stablize the breathing and kick the right leg upward 25 times. Then do the same with the left leg (Fig. 128). Repeat the movements 25 to 50 times.

6. Kicking in an Arched Position

1) Inhale and support the body with the four limbs. Raise the body and make the forehead approach both knees. Lift the right knee to meet the forehead.

2) Exhale and contract the muscles of the buttocks. Raise the head and stretch the right leg to the ceiling. Don't stop inhaling and bring the forehead and the right knee together. Kick again. The movement should be quick and continuous, violence should be avoided. Do this several times (Fig. 129). Practise with each leg 10 to 25 times.

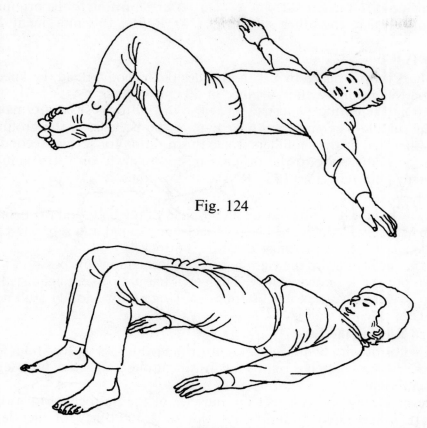

Fig. 124

Fig. 125

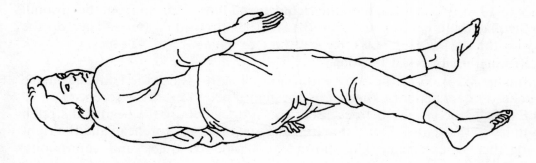

Fig. 126

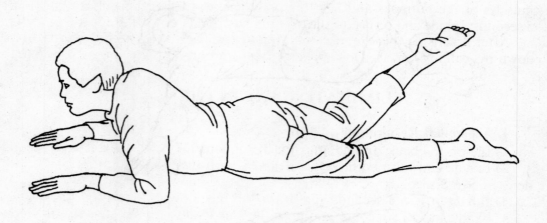

Fig. 127

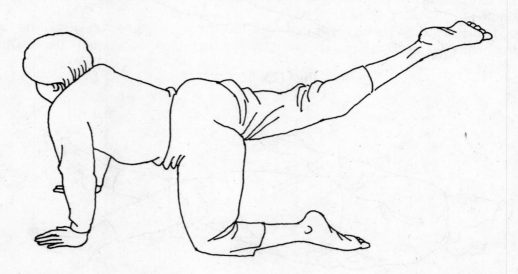

Fig. 128

7. Folding-up

1) Kneel down with the hands at the sides and palms slightly touching the sides of the legs.

2) Inhale and keep the trunk and femur on the same line. Contract tightly the muscles of the buttocks and lean the body backward. Remain in this position for 5 seconds. Inhale and return to the original position (Fig.130). Repeat 5 to 15 times.

After practising this exercise, one should regulate the breathing and try to calm down by walking slowly. Don't sit down before normal breathing is restored.

ELIMINATING FAT IN THE WAIST

1. Abdominal Respiration

1) Lie on the back. Inhale, making the abdomen full of air in 1 to 4 seconds.

2) Exhale and raise both feet 45 degrees, with the toes straight. This should be done in 5 to 8 seconds.

3) Inhale in 1 to 4 seconds and lower the feet slowly.

4) Exhale in 5 to 8 seconds and raise the feet 45 degrees. Practise this movement 8 times every day on an empty stomach.

2. Twisting Massage

Keep the body close to a brush and twist the body to get a rubbing stimulation. Direct stimulation to the subcutaneous fat can lead to tension in the muscles. Also this movement can generally cause consumption of thermal energy and result in slimness.

1) Stand straight with separated feet. Put the brush in the height of the waist. Brush the waist while twisting the body, twisting in each direction more than 20 times.

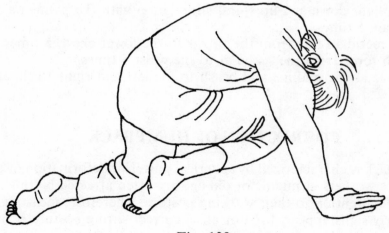

Fig. 129

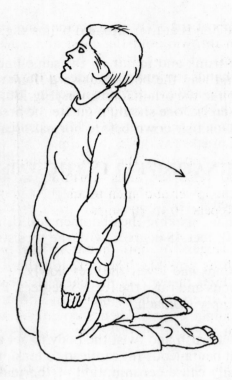

Fig. 130

2) Brush the back 20 times while twisting the body.

3. Cosmetics by *Jingluo* Stimulation

1) Perform light down-and-up spiral stimulation with the palms on the Foot-Kidney Meridian, 5 times.

2) Rub the meridian line from the thighs to the lower chest, 5 times.

3) Rub with force from the scapular to the waist 5 times.

Take this line as the midline and brush to the left and right 10 times on each side.

CORRECTION OF HUMPBACK

The humpback is characterized by spherical posterior deformation of the spinal coloumn. Office workers at middle or old age are often affected by this syndrome if they pay little attention to their working posture. Therefore, measures must be taken when early signs appear. First of all, a correct sitting posture is important. In addition, the following exercises can be practised to correct deformation.

1. Exercises in Bed

1) Lie on the back. Support the body with occiput and both elbows and throw out the chest. Inhale when throwing out the chest and exhale when lowering the body. Repeat 10 to 20 times.

2) Lie on the back with hands resting on the sides of the body. Raise the head and shoulders. Inhale when raising and exhale when lowering. Repeat 10 to 20 times.

3) Lie on the back, with the hands resting on the sides of the body. Raise the head and shoulders, remaining in this position for 10 seconds. Then lower the body. Repeat again after a short break. Do this 5 to 8 times.

4) Lie face downwards, supporting the body with both arms and toes. First, contract the abdomen and raise the anus, forming an arch. Then lower the buttocks, waist and make the lower abdomen touch the bed. At last, raise the head and throw out the chest. Repeat 10 to 20 times.

2. Standing Exercises

1) Put the interlaced fingers of both hands at the back of the neck and close both elbows as much as possible. Then expand them outward and vibrate backward slightly. Meanwhile, throw out the chest. Repeat 10 to 20 times.

2) Put the interlaced fingers of both hands at the back of the neck and bend the waist to the maximal extent. Then straighten the waist and raise the head to the maximal extent, so as to increase the activities of the spinal column. Repeat 10 to 20 times.

3) Raise the arms to the shoulder height in front of the body with palms down and clench the hands. Do the chest-expanding exercise and raise the head, contract the abdomen and throw out the chest at the same time. Repeat 10 to 20 times.

4) Cross the hands, extend the waist and throw out the chest rhythmically, following your inhalation. Exhale when returning to the original position.

The above movements should be done twice a day, 10 to 15 minutes each time. Generally, good results can be achieved in 3 to 6 months.

ELIMINATION OF DOUBLE CHINS

Double chin, an annoying problem, mainly results from decreased elasticity of the muscles and from accumulation of fats due to aging or lack of physical exercise. The following exercises can improve this condition and firm up the relaxed muscles after several weeks' practice.

1. Moving the Jaws

1) Respire twice. Shrug the shoulders upwards as far as possible, until the shoulders almost touch the ears. Raise the chin upward and try to make the back of the head approach the shoulders.

2) Turn the head slowly to one side then to the other side, each side 5 times.

3) Keep the shoulders in a shrugging position and turn the head clockwise. Repeat 5 times. Then do the same counterclockwise.

4) Relax and restore the shoulders in natural position. Then respire twice.

5) Relax the shoulders and repeat the movement.

2. Touching the Shoulders with the Lower Chin and Ears

1) Raise the lower lip to cover the upper lip. Tighten the muscles of the lower chin, being careful not to use strength from the lips or the mouths.

2) Keep the lips in the above position. Touch the left shoulder first with the lower chin and then with the left ear. Do this 5 times before changing to the other side.

3) Repeat the movement in items 1) and 2).

4) Relax and respire twice.

3. Tongue Pressure

1) Raise the lower chin several centimeters and close the teeth naturally.

2) Prop the lower chin with the back of the right hand and put the index finger on the Adam's apple.

3) Prop the lower gum with the tip of tongue and support the lower chin with the back of the right hand to increase resistance. Increase the pressure of the tongue tip to the lower gum for 6 seconds. When the pressure reaches the maximum, hold this position for another 6 seconds.

4) Decrease the pressure slowly and relax. Breathe deeply twice. Repeat the exercise twice.

4. Vacuum Inhalation

1) Respire twice. Keep the teeth in a natural position. Project the lower chin upwards until the muscles of the neck become tight.

2) Close the lips tightly. Keep the movement of the respiration with the muscles of the neck very tight for 10 seconds. This action is not taking in the air, but just tightening the muscles of the neck with the movement of respiration.

Relax and respire three times. Repeat the exercise again.

5. Raising the Lower Chin

1) Raise the lower chin, project it a little forward and open the mouth as wide as possible.

2) Raise the lower chin slowly with the force of the lower chin and muscles of the neck only and keep the head unmoved.

3) Cover the upper lip with the lower lip and hold the upper teeth with the lower teeth. Try hard to touch the nose with the lower lip, holding the breath.

4) Relax. Then do the above exercises 10 times.

6. Closing the Teeth Swiftly

1) Raise the head until the muscles of the neck are tightened. Stick out the lower chin.

2) Keep the head unmoved and open the mouth as wide as possible.

3) Keep the head unmoved and the lower chin projected. Close the teeth slightly and then open them again. Do the quick closing and opening 10 times. Then relax and respire twice. This movement should be repeated 10 times.

7. Leaning Back the Head and Exerting Tongue Pressure

1) Project the lower chin and closely lean the occipital bone toward the back. Keep the teeth in a natural position and cover the upper lip with the lower one with the force of the muscles of the lower chin.

2) Prop the tip of the tongue against the lower part of the gum at the lower incisors. Breathe with the nose. Increase the pressure for 8 seconds until the maximum pressure is being exerted by the tongue. Hold this pressure for over 8 seconds.

3) Relax and respire twice before doing this exercise again.

Women with double chins are sure to get good effects if they persist in practising these exercises.

EXERCISES FOR PUERPERAL RESTORATION

Women who have given birth to a child all hope that their body may look like it did in their maiden life. This is possible if one practises the exercises for puerperal restoration. A brief introduction of these exercises is as follows:

1. Stand with the arms raising up forcefully, or perform sit-ups, or stretch the arms backwards when sitting on a chair without a back.

2. Stand straight and stretch the arms downwards until they touch the ground. Or, lie on the back, get the body up with the hands holding the head and then raise both feet together or the feet alternately, forming an angle of 90 degrees. Or do frog kicks while sitting on a chair.

3. Stand straight and raise both elbows, turning the upper part of the body rightward and leftward while keeping the lower part unmoved. Or, sit on a chair, twist the waist with the hands holding the head.

Generally, one month after beginning this exercise, the waist measurement will lessen about 3 cm on average.

图书在版编目 (CIP) 数据

中国家庭保健实用气功: 英文/金策等编著.

—北京: 外文出版社, 1995

ISBN 7 – 119 – 00070 – 5

Ⅰ. 中… Ⅱ. 金… Ⅲ. ①家庭保健 – 中国 – 英文 ②气功疗法
– 中国 – 英文 Ⅳ. ①R161②R247.4

中国版本图书馆 CIP 数据核字 (95) 第 09627 号

中国家庭保健实用气功

金 策 胡樟桂 金振华 编著

*

©外文出版社

外文出版社出版

(中国北京百万庄路 24 号)

邮政编码 100037

北京外文印刷厂印刷

中国国际图书贸易总公司发行

(中国北京车公庄西路 35 号)

北京邮政信箱第 399 号 邮政编码 100044

1996 年 (16 开) 第一版

(英)

ISBN 7 – 119 – 00070 – 5 /R·121(外)

06880

14 – E – 2988S